The Black Death

The Great Mortality of 1348–1350

A BRIEF HISTORY WITH DOCUMENTS

Second Edition

John Aberth

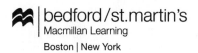
bedford/st.martin's
Macmillan Learning
Boston | New York

For Bedford/St. Martin's

Vice President, Editorial, Macmillan Learning Humanities: Edwin Hill
Publisher for History: Michael Rosenberg
Acquiring Editor for History: Laura Arcari
Director of Development for History: Jane Knetzger
Developmental Editor: Melanie McFadyen
History Marketing Manager: Melissa Famiglietti
Production Editor: Lidia MacDonald-Carr
Production Coordinator: Carolyn Quimby
Director of Rights and Permissions: Hilary Newman
Permissions Associate: Michael McCarty
Permissions Manager: Kalina Ingham
Cover Design: William Boardman
Cover Photo: Black Death at Tournai, 1349 / Le Muisit, Gilles (1272–1352) /
    Bibliotheque Royale de Belgique, Brussels, Belgium / Bridgeman Images
Project Management: Books By Design, Inc.
Cartographer: Mapping Specialists, Ltd.
Composition: Achorn International, Inc.
Printing and Binding: LSC Communications

Copyright © 2017, 2005 by Bedford/St. Martin's.

All rights reserved. No part of this book may be reproduced, stored in a retrieval system, or transmitted in any form or by any means, electronic, mechanical, photocopying, recording, or otherwise, except as may be expressly permitted by the applicable copyright statutes or in writing by the Publisher.

Manufactured in the United States of America.

1   0   9   8   7
f   e   d   c

For information, write: Bedford/St. Martin's, 75 Arlington Street, Boston, MA 02116
    (617-399-4000)

ISBN 978-1-319-04887-7

Acknowledgments

Acknowledgments and copyrights appear on the same page as the text and art selections they cover; these acknowledgments and copyrights constitute an extension of the copyright page.

Foreword

The Bedford Series in History and Culture is designed so that readers can study the past as historians do.

The historian's first task is finding the evidence. Documents, letters, memoirs, interviews, pictures, movies, novels, or poems can provide facts and clues. Then the historian questions and compares the sources. There is more to do than in a courtroom, for hearsay evidence is welcome, and the historian is usually looking for answers beyond act and motive. Different views of an event may be as important as a single verdict. How a story is told may yield as much information as what it says.

Along the way the historian seeks help from other historians and perhaps from specialists in other disciplines. Finally, it is time to write, to decide on an interpretation and how to arrange the evidence for readers.

Each book in this series contains an important historical document or group of documents, each document a witness from the past and open to interpretation in different ways. The documents are combined with some element of historical narrative — an introduction or a biographical essay, for example — that provides students with an analysis of the primary source material and important background information about the world in which it was produced.

Each book in the series focuses on a specific topic within a specific historical period. Each provides a basis for lively thought and discussion about several aspects of the topic and the historian's role. Each is short enough (and inexpensive enough) to be a reasonable one-week assignment in a college course. Whether as classroom or personal reading, each book in the series provides firsthand experience of the challenge — and fun — of discovering, recreating, and interpreting the past.

Lynn Hunt
David W. Blight
Bonnie G. Smith

Preface

The Black Death, or plague, of 1348–1350 is considered by most historians to be the defining event of the late Middle Ages, one that brought in its train a whole host of seismic impacts upon society and culture. This new edition of primary sources has been updated in order to allow students to better understand and appreciate the myriad and wide-ranging effects that the Black Death had on Europe and Southwest Asia. As in the first edition, this collection addresses in separate chapters the geographical origins, symptoms, and transmission of the plague, as well as its medical, social, economic, religious, psychological, and artistic repercussions.

The introduction, Part One, has been revised to include a new section on the "plague denial" controversy, which has been a major focus of Black Death studies in recent years. In particular, this section addresses the latest developments in paleomicrobiology, which have managed to isolate, positively identify, and even reconstruct the genome or DNA of *Yersinia pestis*, the bacterium responsible for plague, from samples taken from Black Death victims in mass grave pits. This holds the promise of finally bringing closure to this debate and allowing researchers to focus their attention on more productive pursuits.

Part Two, The Documents, retains its focus on the first outbreak of the Black Death in 1348–1350. A host of new documents have been added to reflect the latest trends in Black Death research or to include new sources that have come to light. For example, a new chapter—Chapter 7, Environmental Explanations and Responses—has been added that addresses how the Black Death changed medieval people's perception of the environment and of the natural world. Included in this chapter are an excerpt from the *History of the Plague* by the Piacenzan chronicler Gabriele de Mussis, Konrad of Megenberg's explanation of how the plague was caused by earthquakes, and the plague ordinances enacted by the city of Pistoia in Italy. In Chapter 6, a Middle Dutch flagellant scroll is here presented in English translation for the first time;

this unique source was produced and used by the flagellants themselves as part of their ritual or ceremonies, thus giving us a glimpse into the flagellant movement unfiltered by the (usually hostile) perspectives of contemporary chroniclers. In the "Poison Conspiracy" section (formerly the "Jewish Pogroms"), a series of replies to Strasbourg's interrogatory about the Jews allows us to trace how the poison conspiracy evolved and spread by word of mouth or by letter from town to town throughout the Savoy and the German kingdom. Also included in this chapter are Jean de Fayt's "Sermon on the Flagellants" preached before the pope at Avignon and André Benedict's letter to the jurors of Gerona concerning the proceedings against suspected poison conspirators in Languedoc. Several new images relating to the "plague saints," St. Sebastian and St. Roch, have been added to Chapter 8, The Artistic Response. A new selection from, and translation of, Abū Ja'far Ahmad Ibn Khātima's "Description and Remedy for Escaping the Plague," relating to symptoms and transmission of the Black Death, has been added to Chapter 2. Chapter 3, Medical Responses, includes an expanded version of Gentile da Foligno's "Short Casebook" from 1348.

To facilitate students' understanding and interpretation of each selection, the general and chapter introductions outline the medieval context within which the sources were created, as well as modern historiographical concerns. Such background material includes the historical significance and impact of the Black Death, how contemporaries viewed and debated the event, the circumstances of and approaches to their recording of it, how interpretations of the plague have changed over time, and what the current scholarly consensus—if there is one—may be on its various aspects. The document headnotes give more specific context concerning the author and date of composition, and gloss notes explain unfamiliar terms or concepts in the documents. The volume closes with a Chronology, revised Questions for Consideration, and an updated Selected Bibliography arranged by chapter topic for further reading.

A NOTE ABOUT THE TEXT AND TRANSLATIONS

Most documents in this collection were written in Latin, the universal learned language of western Europe during the Middle Ages. However, by the late medieval period, vernacular languages were coming into vogue, and these survive in a growing number of sources. Thus, several other languages are also represented: Italian, German, French, Spanish, and English, as well as Greek and Arabic used in the eastern Mediterranean.

ACKNOWLEDGMENTS

Translation of this number and variety of sources would not have been possible without substantial help. For translations of German and Italian sources, I have availed myself of the services of Thomas Huber and Aubrey Threlkeld; and for Dutch, of Bertus Brokamp. I am also grateful to Walid Saleh for assistance with the Arabic source of Ibn al-Khatīb, although I am fully responsible for this translation. I would also like to thank Professor Walter Simons of Dartmouth College for providing me with the published article of the Middle Dutch flagellant scroll in Document 22. I also have benefited from the constructive comments of several reviewers of the manuscript, including Richard Gyug, Fordham University; Erin Jordan, University of Northern Colorado; Timothy Kircher, Guilford College; and Carol Quillen, Rice University. In addition, I must thank the interlibrary loan departments of the University of Vermont and of Middlebury College for their assiduous and timely response to my many requests for documents. The students in my Black Death classes have helped me realize which sources are most useful and interesting for a study of this topic. I would also like to thank the following people from Bedford/St. Martin's for their hard work and assistance in bringing this book to completion: Publisher for History Michael Rosenberg, Acquiring Editor Laura Arcari, Director of Development for History Jane Knetzger, History Marketing Manager Melissa Famiglietti, Editorial Assistant and Developmental Editor Melanie McFadyen, Production Editor Lidia MacDonald-Carr, Cover Designer William Boardman, and Production Coordinator Nancy Benjamin of Books By Design. Above all, I must thank my wife, Laura Hamilton, for putting up so long with a man obsessed with so morbid a subject.

John Aberth

Contents

Map and Illustrations

PART ONE

Introduction: The Black Death in History

> It so happened that in the month of October in the year of our Lord 1347, around the first of that month, twelve Genoese galleys, fleeing our Lord's wrath which came down upon them for their misdeeds, put in at the port of the city of Messina. They brought with them a plague that they carried down to the very marrow of their bones, so that if anyone so much as spoke to them, he was infected with a mortal sickness which brought on an immediate death that he could in no way avoid.[1]

Such is how the Black Death first arrived on the shores of Europe, according to the Sicilian chronicler Michele da Piazza. Within the next two to three years, the epidemic became a pandemic as it spread throughout nearly the entire continent and its islands and wiped out half or more of its population. Although modern students and historians refer to this pandemic as the Black Death, the men and women who experienced the disease never called it by this name. Instead, medieval accounts speak of the "pestilence," the "plague" (from the Latin word *plaga*, meaning "a blow" or "an affliction"), or the "great mortality." The term "the Black Death" was first coined in the sixteenth century and popularized in the nineteenth. Even so, Black Death is now the standard designation for this event, the so-called Second Pandemic of a disease that first afflicted Europe—specifically, the Mediterranean region—between 541 and 750 CE, and struck a third time in China, India, and elsewhere around the world between 1855 and 1959.

THE BLACK DEATH AS HISTORICAL EVENT

The Black Death is a watershed event in history because of the timing, geography, and extent of its appearance. The disease struck at a time when Europe had not known an outbreak of plague since the First Pandemic many centuries earlier. Although a "Great Famine" struck northern Europe between 1315 and 1322, nothing prepared Europeans for the horrendous onslaught of the Black Death. One should never discount the initial shock that the disease caused throughout Europe between 1348 and 1350. One chronicler, Agnolo di Tura of Siena, reported that "so many have died that everyone believes it is the end of the world." And the Black Death returned, albeit with considerably less virulence, almost once a decade throughout the second half of the fourteenth and the entire fifteenth centuries. Plague and other diseases kept Europe's population stagnant or even slightly in decline until well into the early modern period.

The great mortality of 1348–1350 was also wide ranging in its geographical incidence. It affected every country and region in Europe, with the probable exception of Iceland and Finland, whose relative isolation from mercantile contacts may have spared them. The Black Death was therefore a shared experience among medieval Europeans, producing a remarkably similar set of responses. Some European chroniclers were fully aware that they were part of a worldwide phenomenon, which embraced both neighboring regions and lands as far away as China and India. Plague probably began as an *endemic*, that is, a locally confined disease that, once established, is perpetually present in a given area. Such endemic foci of plague are now present on almost every continent, but, based on genetic sampling, it seems that the original endemic focus of plague was in the Tibetan plateau just north of the Himalayan mountains, the so-called roof of the world. Plague then broke out in *epidemics* (that is, diseases occurring in a local population or community) and *pandemics* (worldwide occurrences of disease) when flea, rodent, or human populations spread the disease farther afield through faster, more efficient trade or communication networks. The establishment of the far-flung Mongol Empire by the second half of the thirteenth century linked Asia to Europe in an overland network of mounted armies, postal carriers, and caravans. Once transmitted from its endemic foci in the East, the plague easily made its way across Europe through well-established trade links (Chapter 1).

Finally, the Black Death was unusually potent in the human mortality it caused. Previously, the prevailing view among modern scholars was that the disease carried off roughly a third of Europe's inhabitants during its first and most devastating outbreak, from 1348 to 1350. New research suggests that this estimate must be revised upward to an *average* mortality rate of 50–60 percent.[2] English episcopal registers, which record deaths among the parish clergy within a bishop's diocese and are among the most professionally recorded medieval documents available, yield a mean mortality rate of 45–47 percent. Manorial records, which also survive from England and which register the deaths of a lord's tenants, all point to death rates between roughly 45 and 55 percent. Although fewer records survive on the continent than in England, a variety of documents, including parish registers, tax assessments, household census returns, scribal records, and episcopal registers from France, Italy, and Spain, record national mortality rates ranging from 45 to 60 percent. A 50 percent average mortality rate also would be more in line with what medieval chroniclers wrote about the Black Death. Although we must always approach medieval numerical estimates with caution, as they are prone to exaggeration, these estimates nonetheless testify to the perceived severity of the disease. If "the living were hardly able to bury the dead," as many English chroniclers report, then the death rate—regardless of the exact figure—was high enough to create an intolerable burden.

HISTORICAL SIGNIFICANCE OF THE BLACK DEATH

The ever-higher estimates of plague mortality, and the uncovering of much economic disruption and upheaval on manors behind the façade of recovery,[3] have only added to the importance of the Black Death as an event of great historical significance. It was not always this way. Almost fifty years ago, a collection of essays—*The Black Death: A Turning Point in History?*[4]—indicated just by the question mark in its title that the Black Death's pivotal role in late medieval society, long assumed, was now being challenged. Arguing on the basis of neo-Malthusian economics, which begins with Thomas Malthus's principle that "the power of population is indefinitely greater than the power in the earth to produce subsistence for man," the revisionist historians recast the Black Death as a necessary and long-overdue corrective to an overpopulated Europe.[5] In this view, the disease was not a sudden and violent eruption but an inevitable consequence of a medieval population that had outgrown its capacity to feed itself. Since the mid-1980s, postrevisionist historians have been swinging the pendulum back, restoring the Black Death as a watershed in late medieval history.[6] But even though there is general consensus—based on our firmer grasp of its mortality rate—that the Black Death was the greatest natural disaster in the history of humankind,[7] there is still much room for debate about the *kind* of impacts that it had. Which kinds of impacts were beneficial, and which harmful, and for whom?

For some historians, the Black Death, aside from its horrendous mortality, had mostly positive effects. This has been christened the "silver lining" thesis, which began to take hold in the 1980s and 1990s and has largely held its own until the present day. For these historians, plague provides "proof of humanity's ability to endure even the worst crisis, to rebuild, and to start again."[8] For others, the Black Death represented an opportunity for medieval Europeans to break out of their Malthusian deadlock in terms of the relationship between population and resources, or the land-labor ratio. This then initiated a number of unintended, but beneficial, consequences, including new surpluses of wealth that stimulated economic prosperity; labor-saving innovations in technology; and reform and renewal of late medieval society and culture, particularly in terms of religious and cultural sensibilities, medicine, philosophy, and education.[9]

Nonetheless, one can certainly challenge various aspects of the silver lining thesis and produce a more nuanced picture of its view of plague's mostly positive impacts on late medieval society. For example, the Black Death was not the main driver behind all advances in late medieval technology: The printing press, a device usually credited to the German printer Johannes Gutenberg around 1450, was inspired more by greater literacy and therefore greater appetite for books among Europe's population than by a desire or need to save labor in copying manuscripts by hand.[10] It is also not clear how extensive were the economic benefits conveyed by the Black Death, since only a minority of peasants made their living exclusively from wage labor or had the resources to fully enter the land market.[11] Similar uncertainties surround the claim that the Black Death opened new economic opportunities for women, thus liberating them from the pressure to marry early and have children.[12] The Black Death did inaugurate a new response from doctors to disease—the poison thesis—but this was not necessarily more practical or effective, at least from a modern perspective, than previous responses.[13]

Through all these debates, there remains the simple fact that the Black Death was, indeed, the greatest and most sustained demographic disaster in the history of the world. As a consequence, it makes sense to argue that its broad socioeconomic and cultural impact was correspondingly immense. There can be no question anymore that the Black

Death, with its high cumulative mortality, did beget big changes, and that these changes nudged medieval society into the early modern era.[14] Any attempt to deny or mitigate the importance and large-scale impact of the Black Death, as has been attempted by various schools of historical interpretation, must be judged as doomed to failure.[15]

As the documents that follow demonstrate, plague's effects on late medieval society were extremely varied: medical, social, economic, psychological, religious, and artistic. Although the people of the later Middle Ages had relatively primitive medical technologies, they nonetheless possessed a confident outlook that put even an apocalyptic disaster of the magnitude of the Black Death into the perspective of God's secure and benevolent plan for humankind. The English anchoress and mystic Julian of Norwich, who lived through no fewer than eight national outbreaks of plague, including the one of 1348–1350, and who may have suffered from the disease herself, was yet able to declare that "alle shalle be wele" with the world.[16] Many chroniclers of the plague wrote as if the apocalypse, the end of creation, was at hand, but in medieval eschatology, the apocalypse also signified a new beginning. No longer can scholars afford to dismiss the later Middle Ages as simply an era of decline. Rather, Europe's Renaissance, or "rebirth," was forged in the crucible of its terrible, yet transcendent, ordeal with the Black Death.

THE PLAGUE DENIAL CONTROVERSY

Much of our current knowledge of plague comes from medical researchers and their personal experience in the field of fighting plague in China and India during the early years of the Third Pandemic, around the turn of the twentieth century.[17] These same researchers first gave scientific credence to the theory that the Black Death was to be identified with plague. By the 1970s and 1980s, however, this traditional identification was being called into question by writers with professional expertise in bacteriology and zoology but who had little training in historical research and interpretation.[18] Nonetheless, by the turn of the twenty-first century, plague denial was being enthusiastically taken up by some historians.[19] Their main lines of argument included the following: (1) the Black Death spread too fast and across areas too remotely settled by animals or humans to be bubonic plague; (2) there are too few reports of rat infestations or of outbreaks of the disease among rats in both literary and archaeological artifacts dating to the Black Death for there to be a connection between the two; and (3) the descriptions of symptoms of the Black Death in contemporary chronicles, medical treatises, and other sources are inconsistent with a modern diagnosis of plague.

In the end, the plague denial controversy was settled by some new and rather unusual evidence: centuries-old blood samples from plague victims buried in mass graves, namely, the dental pulp encapsulated in the victims' teeth. Through a technique pioneered by French researchers in the late 1990s, the dental pulp was extracted and then analyzed, revealing the positive identification of the DNA of the plague bacterium *Yersinia pestis* in the remains.[20] (The study of such ancient microorganisms recovered from excavated grave sites is now known as the field of "paleomicrobiology.") Progressively new and better techniques at testing for *Yersinia pestis* DNA in ancient remains yielded more reliable results.[21] Eventually, this effort culminated in the successful reconstruction of a complete genome, or DNA sequence, of a *Yersinia pestis* sample taken from plague victims buried in London's East Smithfield cemetery, dating to the very first outbreak of the Black Death, in 1348–1349.[22] Since the genome shows damage patterns consistent with aging in other ancient samples, this proves that it is medieval, and not contaminated by modern *Yersinia pestis* DNA, as was claimed of earlier paleomicrobiological studies.[23]

Although the evidence indicates that the Black Death was caused by new, unprecedented strains of *Yersinia pestis* that emerged since the First Pandemic of the early Middle Ages, it is also clear that the Black Death strains introduced the world to plague as we know it today. Comparison of medieval and modern strains demonstrates just how few genetic changes, especially in terms of the plasmid responsible for virulence, have accrued to *Yersinia pestis* DNA since the Black Death pandemic of 1348–1350.[24] This means that, as a toxic organism, *Yersinia pestis* has barely changed in the past six and a half centuries and more, remaining as deadly today as it was in the Middle Ages.

Thus far, at least twenty separate paleomicrobiological studies— representing thirty-five grave sites in five different countries dating to both the First and Second Pandemics—have independently confirmed that the Black Death was indeed plague, based on the successful isolation and identification of *Yersinia pestis* DNA from the dental pulp of plague victims. Cumulatively, the data is impressive enough that it has convinced scholars reviewing the evidence that the debate over whether the Black Death is plague is now effectively over.[25]

But some plague deniers still hold out against such a conclusion; indeed, they declared their intention, well before all the paleomicrobiological evidence was in, of disputing, or simply ignoring altogether, whatever results were obtained.[26] Their hard-line position has been aided by the view that the "laboratory construction of plague"—that is, the modern knowledge that plague is caused by the *Yersinia pestis* bacterium, which was discovered by the Swiss bacteriologist Alexandre Yersin in 1894—can never be applied to past epidemics, such as the Black Death, when contemporaries had no awareness of germs. The argument here is that there is an "unbridgeable gap" between modern and premodern plague, and that the criteria of "sameness" have been changed, because in the latter instance, we must rely on subjective evidence, such as descriptions in chronicles and other writings, that reflect the very different views contemporaries had of disease.[27] However, this position has been resoundingly disproven by paleomicrobiology, which has demonstrated that the laboratory construction of plague can, indeed, be applied to the victims of the Black Death, since *Yersinia pestis* can now be isolated from these victims, just like it can be done for modern patients. Nonetheless, plague deniers contend that their original objections automatically invalidate, or at least pose almost irreconcilable caveats to, any evidence adduced to the contrary.[28] Remarkably, this would privilege historical interpretation over scientific fact or proof.

Unfortunately for plague deniers, their original arguments are not so ironclad or invincible as claimed. Hand in hand with the new evidence provided by paleomicrobiology, there has been a critical reexamination— or, one might say, examination, since such scrutiny has rarely been attempted before now—of the case for plague denial.[29] This reexamination has found plague denial's arguments to be profoundly weak and fatally undermined by numerous logical fallacies. Thus, what has been cited as the "insoluble conundrum" between what the science of paleomicrobiology and the historical evidence allegedly say, is really no mystery at all: Both, in fact, confirm conclusively that the Black Death was plague.[30]

One can easily point out the glaring inconsistencies of plague denial by referencing some of the sources contained in this book. For example, as already mentioned, plague deniers claim that the Black Death spread too fast to be bubonic plague—a favorite phrase is that the Black Death spread "almost as quickly" in a day as modern plague spreads in a year.[31] But this falsely equates two separate and distinct phenomena, namely, the spread rate (that is, how fast a disease travels from point A to point B) of human epidemics or pandemics of plague, and the spread rate of epizootics, or outbreaks of the disease among wild rodents. Human epidemics of plague typically spread via "metastatic leaps"—from one site to another, in which plague carriers, namely, rats and their fleas, hitch a ride in human-mediated transport, such as ships (traveling an average of twenty-five miles per day) and cart- or pack-horse caravans (traveling twelve to thirty miles per day).[32] Epizootics, however, typically spread slowly and gradually—anywhere from four to twenty miles per year— by contiguous means, as one infected rodent colony contaminates an adjacent one through the animals' own power.[33] Thus, the circumstances of these two phenomena are not really comparable. (There is almost no evidence for a spread rate of epizootics in medieval times.) Moreover, metastatic leaps are a much more haphazard and unpredictable means of spreading disease than simply tracing a contact from point A to point B.[34] Contemporaries like Konrad of Megenberg (Document 29) and Heinrich of Herford observed this phenomenon when they mentioned how the plague seemed to move "with an accidental or involuntary motion like some bodily form propelled by winds in the airy regions," or like a player "in a game of chess, rising up from one place in which it had raged, [then] passing by an intermediate one without contaminating it to rage in a third, and perchance afterwards going back to the intermediate place" to rage there for the first time.[35]

Arguing from silence in the medieval record is another fallacy committed by plague deniers, when they point to no rats, or not enough of them, to spread bubonic plague during the Black Death.[36] (If a rat died of plague and no one was around to see it, did it cause an epidemic?) Part of the silence may simply be a function of how we look for medieval rats.

Archaeologically, rat bones may be missed by excavators unless they use proper sieving equipment (1–2 mm mesh or smaller) and examine sieved residue under a microscope.[37] Linguistically speaking, there are challenges in that Latin did not distinguish between a rat and a mouse (*mus* doing double duty for both), and vernacular terms for rat were only just coming into use during the late Middle Ages.[38] In addition, the silence on medieval rats may be a reflection of how attuned we are to medieval sources and evidence. Many medieval medical authorities did mention how rats or mice and other vermin "that dwell underground" would flee to the surface and exit their holes just before a plague epidemic, which was taken as a reliable sign to watch for. But, as was typical of most medieval authors, who generally favored ancient authority or tradition over their own empirical observation, these doctors were not describing an actual experience from the Black Death; rather, they were paraphrasing a passage from the *Canon* of the eleventh-century Persian physician Avicenna (Ibn Sīnā).[39] This does not mean that an authentic observation of a medieval rat could not be made: The fifteenth-century Strasbourg physician John of Saxony relates a personal anecdote of how a neighbor's house, where eight children died of bubonic plague in as many days, was inundated with so many rats or mice that the household servants "could not fend them off" and were forced to decamp, leaving "a lamp burning that is [still] there to the present [day]."[40] Surely it is unrealistic to expect medieval authors to observe rats in the same way that we would today: Not even the "rat intelligence staff" deployed by researchers of the Third Pandemic in India were able to easily find rats who died of plague, since typically these animals, when sick, burrowed deep into walls and roofs to escape predation from other rats.[41] The modern expectation that millions of rats would fall from the sky (or at least the roof) and crawl into the streets to die and create an unavoidable spectacle for medieval chroniclers to comment on is more the product of folktale fantasy (such as the Pied Piper of Hamlin) than of reality.[42] Remarkably, the notion still betrays the influence of Avicenna's ideas from nearly a millennium ago.

The fallacy of false equivalence also plagues (pardon the pun) deniers' claims that medieval doctors and chroniclers did not describe the same disease as modern plague.[43] Again, one can ask, is it realistic for them to do so? Certainly, most literary authors, and even professional physicians, of the Middle Ages could not hope to meet the exacting diagnostic standards that we take for granted today. A good example is how many medieval doctors make the striking claim that bubonic swellings appeared in a veritable rainbow of colors, including red, yellow, green, and black.[44] But this is not necessarily anything that doctors actually saw; it is lifted straight out of the *Prognostics*, attributed to the ancient Greek physician Hippocrates (460–370 BCE).[45] Once again, we should not expect medieval authors to make reliable, firsthand observations when they seem to privilege time-honored authorities and traditions.[46] This is also not to say, however, that some medieval doctors did not speak from experience. One who did so (which included coming down with two buboes on his groin) was the fifteenth-century Catalan physician Blasius of Barcelona; he states emphatically that the colors of red, blue, and black "are very rarely to be found in glandular swellings."[47] Another doctor who lived through the Black Death, the Moorish physician from Almería, Abū Ja'far Ahmad Ibn Khātima, is likewise known for his empirical observations, which include the case histories of his patients. His description of the "three forms" of the disease reads almost like a modern clinical diagnosis of bubonic, pneumonic, and septicemic plague (Document 6). Plague deniers fail to be discriminating in their use of historical evidence, or to evaluate it based on context.

Given the overwhelming verdict of the paleomicrobiological evidence, the identification of the Black Death with plague has now attained the status of scientific fact. Those who continue to deny this reality risk being relegated to the fringe of Black Death scholarship. It is time for historians to move on to a more productive pursuit of the remaining mysteries and conundrums surrounding the Black Death, of which there is still an abundance.

STUDYING MEDIEVAL SOURCES

Medieval chroniclers of the Black Death had a growing awareness that they were recording for posterity. One eyewitness, John Clynn, a Franciscan friar from Kilkenny, Ireland, who would himself die as he memorialized the plague's march across his land, writes movingly at the end of his contribution for 1348 and 1349 to the *Annalium Hiberniae Chronicon* (*Yearly Chronicle of Ireland*):

> But I, Brother John Clynn, of the order of the Friars Minor of the convent of Kilkenny, have written in this book these notable events which occurred in my time, which I uncovered by my own authority or by a correspondent worthy of belief. And in order that noteworthy deeds may not perish with time and fade from the memory of future generations, I, seeing these many misfortunes and almost the whole world enmeshed in malignity, waiting among the dead for death that yet may come, have set down in writing what I have heard and examined as true. And so that the writing may not perish with the writer, and at the same time the work may not cease with the workman, I bequeath the parchment for continuing the work, if by chance a man, or anyone descended from Adam, should remain behind in the future who can escape this pestilence and continue the work I have begun.[48]

Clynn tells us exactly how he acquired his information and what his motives are in committing it to "parchment." But some early Renaissance writers on the plague went beyond eyewitness testimony and the examination of sources. For Giovanni Boccaccio (Document 12) and Francesco Petrarch (Document 11), the Black Death seems to have stirred a newfound realization that the author was a subjective observer of events, rather than the moral certitude that he was recording a history already written by God's salvation plan for the human race, as was typical of most medieval chroniclers. In this sense, the Black Death may have been a turning point in historical writing.[49]

It may be confusing to modern readers that medieval authors gave equal credence to events and explanations with a supernatural or divine origin as to those grounded in what today we would call science. For them, there was no difference between the two. This was especially true with regard to the Black Death, because most medieval authorities assumed that it was ultimately caused by God's will intervening in human affairs as an act of chastisement for humankind's wickedness and sin. Even medical experts, like Gui de Chauliac, physician to the pope, and members of the faculty of medicine at the University of Paris, when attempting to give "scientific" explanations of the disease, frankly admitted that medicine could not help when the plague came from the will of the Almighty (Document 7). Authors like Louis Sanctus (Document 4), who describe the origins of the disease in apocalyptic language, may simply be referencing the Old or New Testament—particularly those sections describing plagues in the book of Exodus or the book of Revelation—to convey the awe-inspiring impact of the disaster. However, it is entirely possible that they are conveying reports from the East of environmental catastrophes—such as earthquakes, droughts, or floods—which may have actually occurred, precipitating the influx of plague-bearing rodents into areas of human habitation.

These documents make it obvious that medieval people had a completely different outlook on both life and death from our own. Yet there is also much that is similar. Then, as now, parents and children were tormented by the loss of family members and scarred by abandonment in time of crisis. Like present-day victims of incurable diseases, who are willing to experiment with "cocktails" of experimental drugs, medieval patients desperately sought remedies for the plague, including recipes containing chopped-up snakes or ground-up gold and emeralds. And, as in the twentieth century, fourteenth-century Europeans, facing what seemed to be an imminent collapse of their civilization, found convenient scapegoats in the Jews. Understanding medieval people requires an effort to bridge the gulf of time separating us from the past, as well as to relive their experience in the present. Above all, students of medieval history must learn to read and view records and artifacts through medieval eyes. Only in this way can we begin to comprehend what it was like to experience the Black Death.

NOTES

[1] Michele da Piazza, *Cronaca*, ed. Antonino Giuffrida (Palermo: ILA Palma, 1980), 82.

[2] Ole J. Benedictow, *The Black Death, 1346–1353: The Complete History* (Woodbridge, Suffolk: Boydell Press, 2004), 245–384; John Aberth, *From the Brink of the Apocalypse: Confronting Famine, War, Plague, and Death in the Later Middle Ages*, 2nd ed. (London: Routledge, 2010), 89–94.

[3] David Stone, "The Black Death and Its Immediate Aftermath: Crisis and Change in the Fenland Economy, 1346–1353," in *Town and Countryside in the Age of the Black Death: Essays in Honour of John Hatcher*, ed. Mark Bailey and Sidney Rigby (Turnhout, Belgium: Brepols, 2012), 213–44.

[4]*The Black Death: A Turning Point in History?*, ed. William M. Bowsky (New York: Holt, Rinehart and Winston, 1971).

[5]The original quote is from Thomas Robert Malthus, *First Essay on Population, 1798* (London: Macmillan, 1926), 12. The main apostle of neo-Malthusianism is widely considered to be the Cambridge historian Michael Moissey Postan, but other adherents include Georges Duby, Emmanuel Le Roy Ladurie, and Wilhelm Abel. For accessible collections of their works, see M. M. Postan, *Essays on Medieval Agriculture and General Problems of the Medieval Economy* (Cambridge: Cambridge University Press, 1973); Wilhelm Abel, *Agricultural Fluctuations in Europe from the Thirteenth to the Twentieth Centuries*, trans. Olive Ordish (London: Methuen, 1980); Georges Duby, *Rural Economy and Country Life in the Medieval West*, trans. C. Postan (Columbia: University of South Carolina Press, 1968); Emmanuel Le Roy Ladurie, "A Reply to Robert Brenner," in *The Brenner Debate: Agrarian Class Structure and Economic Development in Pre-industrial Europe*, ed. T. H. Aston and C. H. E. Philpin (Cambridge: Cambridge University Press, 1985), 101–6.

[6]The postrevisionist argument is mainly put forward in David Herlihy, *The Black Death and the Transformation of the West*, ed. Samuel K. Cohn Jr. (Cambridge, Mass.: Harvard University Press, 1997), 39–81; Samuel K. Cohn Jr., *The Black Death Transformed: Disease and Culture in Early Renaissance Europe* (London and New York: Arnold and Oxford University Press, 2003), 223–52. Herlihy's posthumously published book is based on lectures he originally gave at the University of Maine in 1985. See Herlihy, *Black Death*, p. 1.

[7]For example, see Paul Freedman, *The Origins of Peasant Servitude in Medieval Catalonia* (Cambridge: Cambridge University Press, 1991), 156 ("the most cataclysmic event in medieval European history"); D. G. Watts, "The Black Death in Dorset and Hampshire," in *The Black Death in Wessex* (*The Hatcher Review*, 5, 1998), 28 (the "greatest human disaster in the recorded history of southern England"); Benedictow, *The Black Death*, 3 ("greatest-ever demographic disaster"); Paula Arthur, "The Black Death and Mortality: A Reassessment," in *Fourteenth Century England, VI*, ed. Chris Given-Wilson (Woodbridge, Suffolk: Boydell Press, 2010), 9 ("England's worst natural disaster in history"); Mark Bailey, "Introduction: England in the Age of the Black Death," in *Town and Countryside in the Age of the Black Death: Essays in Honour of John Hatcher* (Turnhout, Belgium: Brepols, 2012), xx ("the greatest disaster in documented human history"); Stone, "The Black Death," 213 ("one of the most cataclysmic episodes in history").

[8]Faye Marie Getz, "Black Death and the Silver Lining: Meaning, Continuity, and Revolutionary Change in Histories of Medieval Plague," *Journal of the History of Biology* 24 (1991): 288.

[9]Herlihy, *Black Death and the Transformation of the West*, 1, 4, and *passim*; Samuel K. Cohn Jr., *The Cult of Remembrance and the Black Death: Six Renaissance Cities in Central Italy* (Baltimore, Md.: Johns Hopkins University Press, 1992); Cohn, *Black Death Transformed*; and Samuel K. Cohn Jr., "Triumph over Plague: Culture and Memory after the Black Death," in *Care for the Here and the Hereafter: Memoria, Art and Ritual in the Middle Ages*, ed. T. Van Bueren (Turnhout, Belgium: Brepols, 2005).

[10]A. Derville, "L'alphabétisation du peuple à la fin du Moyen Age," *Revue du Nord* 26 (1984): 759–72; J. A. H. Moran, *The Growth of English Schooling, 1340–1548: Learning, Literacy, and Laicization in Pre-Reformation York Diocese* (Princeton, N.J.: Princeton University Press, 1985); Lucien Febvre and Henri-Jean Martin, *The Coming of the Book: The Impact of Printing, 1450–1800* (London: Verso, 1997); Elizabeth L. Eisenstein, *The Printing Revolution of Early Modern Europe*, 2nd rev. ed. (Cambridge: Cambridge University Press, 2005).

[11]Perhaps the two articles that best represent either side of this debate are John Hatcher, "Unreal Wages: Long-Run Living Standards and the 'Golden Age' of the Fifteenth Century," in *Commercial Activity, Markets and Entrepreneurs in the Middle Ages: Essays in Honour of Richard Britnell*, ed. Ben Dodds and Christian D. Liddy (Woodbridge, Suffolk: Boydell Press, 2011), 1–24; Christopher Dyer, "A Golden Age Rediscovered: Labourers'

Wages in the Fifteenth Century," in *Money, Prices and Wages: Essays in Honour of Professor Nicholas Mayhew*, ed. Martin Allen and D'Maris Coffman (Basingstoke, Hampshire: Palgrave Macmillan, 2015), 180–95.

[12]The case for expanded employment opportunities for women is made especially by P. J. P. Goldberg, *Women, Work, and Life Cycle in a Medieval Economy: Women in York and Yorkshire, c. 1300–1520* (Oxford: Clarendon Press, 1992), 336–37, 345, 352, 361; and Caroline Barron, "The 'Golden Age' of Women in Medieval London," in *Medieval Women in Southern England* (Reading Medieval Studies, 15, 1989), 35–58. For a rebuttal of this argument, see Mark Bailey, "Demographic Decline in Late Medieval England: Some Thoughts on Recent Research," *Economic History Review* 49 (1996): 9–14.

[13]The case for medieval doctors evincing a newfound empiricism in response to the Black Death is made by Samuel Cohn in *Black Death Transformed*, 67–68, and Samuel K. Cohn Jr., "The Black Death: End of a Paradigm," *American Historical Review* 107 (2002): 707–10. Cohn's position is criticized by Ole J. Benedictow, *What Disease Was Plague? On the Controversy over the Microbiological Identity of Plague Epidemics of the Past* (Leiden: Brill, 2010), 340–41, 346–48, 351, 358–59, 362, 365. See also John Aberth, *Doctoring the Black Death: Europe's Late Medieval Medical Response to Epidemic Disease*, forthcoming with Rowman and Littlefield.

[14]Benedictow, *Black Death*, 387–88.

[15]Mainly it has been the neo-Malthusian, neo-Marxist, and *Annales* schools of interpretation that have attempted to downplay or mitigate the importance of the Black Death. See John Hatcher and Mark Bailey, *Modelling the Middle Ages: The History and Theory of England's Economic Development* (Oxford: Oxford University Press, 2001), 18–20, 26, 57, 176–82; Robert Brenner, "Agrarian Class Structure and Economic Development in Preindustrial Europe," in *The Brenner Debate*, 267–68, 97*n*, and 270.

[16]Julian of Norwich, *Revelations of Divine Love*, long text, chapter 27.

[17]The findings of the Indian Plague Research Commission were published annually in the *Journal of Hygiene* from 1906 to 1937 and are available online at www.ncbi.nlm.nih .gov/pmc/journals/336. Investigations resulting from the pneumonic plague outbreaks in Manchuria in 1910–1911 and 1920–1921 were published by Dr. Wu Liande, head of the North Manchurian Plague Prevention Service, and are conveniently summarized in his *Treatise on Pneumonic Plague* (Geneva: League of Nations Health Organization, 1926).

[18]J. F. D. Shrewsbury, *A History of Bubonic Plague in the British Isles* (Cambridge: Cambridge University Press, 1970); Graham Twigg, *The Black Death: A Biological Reappraisal* (New York: Schocken Books, 1984).

[19]Susan Scott and Christopher J. Duncan, *Biology of Plagues: Evidence from Historical Populations* (Cambridge: Cambridge University Press, 2001); Susan Scott and Christopher J. Duncan, *Return of the Black Death: The World's Greatest Serial Killer* (Chichester, UK: Wiley, 2004); Cohn, "Black Death: End of a Paradigm," 703–38; Cohn, *Black Death Transformed*; Samuel K. Cohn Jr., "Epidemiology of the Black Death and Successive Waves of Plague," in *Pestilential Complexities: Understanding Medieval Plague*, ed. Vivian Nutton (*Medical History Supplement*, 27, 2008), 74–100; Samuel K. Cohn Jr., "The Historian and the Laboratory: The Black Death Disease," in *The Fifteenth Century, XII: Society in an Age of Plague*, ed. Linda Clark and Carole Rawcliffe (Woodbridge, Suffolk: Boydell and Brewer, 2013), 195–212.

[20]Michel Drancourt et al., "Detection of 400-Year-Old *Yersinia pestis* DNA in Human Dental Pulp: An Approach to the Diagnosis of Ancient Septicemia," *Proceedings of the National Academy of Sciences* 95 (1998): 12637–40.

[21]By 2007, the PCR (polymerase chain reaction) technique had been replaced by an F1 antigen dipstick assay and then by targeted enrichment and high-throughput DNA sequencing, which allowed for accurate testing of large numbers of degraded or fragmented DNA samples. These new techniques have yielded positive *Yersinia pestis* DNA test results in nearly all samples, instead of just one or two by the old PCR method. See Raffaella Bianucci et al., "Technical Note: A Rapid Diagnostic Test Detects Plague in Ancient Human

Remains: An Example of the Interaction between Archeological and Biological Approaches (Southeastern France, 16th–18th Centuries)," *American Journal of Physical Anthropology* 136 (2008): 361–67; Verena J. Schuenemann et al., "Targeted Enrichment of Ancient Pathogens Yielding the pPCP1 Plasmid of *Yersinia pestis* from Victims of the Black Death," *Proceedings of the National Academy of Sciences* 108 (2011): 746; Thi-Nguyen-Ny Tran et al., "High Throughput, Multiplexed Pathogen Detection Authenticates Plague Waves in Medieval Venice, Italy," *PLoS One* 6 (2011): online, e16735; J. L. Bolton, "Looking for *Yersinia pestis*: Scientists, Historians and the Black Death," in *The Fifteenth Century, XII: Society in an Age of Plague*, ed. Linda Clark and Carole Rawcliffe (Woodbridge, Suffolk: Boydell and Brewer, 2013), 22–25.

[22]Schuenemann et al., "Targeted Enrichment of Ancient Pathogens," 746–52; Kirsten I. Bos et al., "A Draft Genome of *Yersinia pestis* from Victims of the Black Death," *Nature* 478 (2011): 506–10.

[23]Schuenemann et al., "Targeted Enrichment of Ancient Pathogens," 746–51; Bos et al., "A Draft Genome of *Yersinia pestis*," 506. Critics include Cohn, *Black Death Transformed*, 248; Alan Cooper and Hendrik N. Poinar, "Ancient DNA: Do It Right or Not at All," *Science* 18 (2000): 1139; J. W. Wood and S. N. DeWitte-Aviña, "Was the Black Death Yersinial Plague?" *The Lancet: Infectious Diseases* 3 (2003): 327–28; Thomas P. Gilbert et al., "Absence of *Yersinia pestis*–specific DNA in Human Teeth from Five European Excavations of Putative Plague Victims," *Microbiology* 150 (2004): 341–54.

[24]Schuenemann et al., "Targeted Enrichment of Ancient Pathogens," 746, 749, 751; Bos et al., "A Draft Genome of *Yersinia pestis*," 506–9; Kirsten I. Bos et al., "*Yersinia pestis*: New Evidence for an Old Infection," *PLoS One* 7 (2012): online, e49803; Stephanie Haensch et al., "Distinct Clones of *Yersinia pestis* Caused the Black Death," *PLoS Pathogens* 6 (2010): online, e1001134.

[25]Lester K. Little, "Plague Historians in Lab Coats," *Past and Present* 213 (2011): 280; Bolton, "Looking for *Yersinia pestis*," 25–26, 28, 36. While acknowledging the conclusiveness of the paleomicrobiological evidence in proving that *Yersinia pestis* was the cause of the Black Death, both Little and Bolton nonetheless still acknowledge the validity of revisionist arguments such as those made by Samuel Cohn, but without subjecting these to any critical analysis or review.

[26]Scott and Duncan, *Return of the Black Death*, 185–90; Cohn, "Epidemiology of the Black Death," 100; Cohn, "Historian and the Laboratory," 196–97, 212.

[27]Andrew Cunningham, "Transforming Plague: The Laboratory and the Identity of Infectious Disease," in *The Laboratory Revolution in Medicine*, ed. Andrew Cunningham and Perry Williams (Cambridge: Cambridge University Press, 1992), 242.

[28]In 2013, Cohn wrote that "isolation of the pathogen alone cannot resolve what was the Black Death disease," owing to the allegedly "extreme" or "extraordinary" differences between the medieval and modern occurrences of plague that he himself identified. See Cohn, "Historian and the Laboratory," 196–97, 212.

[29]Benedictow, *What Disease Was Plague?* The fact that this exhaustive review runs to more than 700 pages indicates how much daunting effort is required to fully rebut all of the arguments that have been made by various scholars for plague denial.

[30]Bolton, "Looking for *Yersinia pestis*," 28. Of course, historical evidence, and even paleomicrobiological data, can be interpreted differently to suit a given agenda. But I would suggest that Bolton accepts too uncritically the arguments made by Cohn and other plague deniers.

[31]Cohn, "Black Death: End of a Paradigm," 712; Cohn, *Black Death Transformed*, 109–11; Cohn, "Epidemiology of the Black Death," 78; Cohn, "Historian and the Laboratory," 201–2; Twigg, *Black Death*, 131–46; Scott and Duncan, *Biology of Plagues*, 358.

[32]Benedictow, *Black Death*, 229–31; Benedictow, *What Disease Was Plague?*, 173, 187; Wendy R. Childs, "Moving Around," in *A Social History of England, 1200–1500*, ed. Rosemary Horrox and W. Mark Ormrod (Cambridge: Cambridge University Press, 2006), 261.

[33]Cohn, "Black Death: End of a Paradigm," 712, 52*n*; Cohn, "Historian and the Laboratory," 201; Twigg, *Black Death*, 139. Almost all this evidence concerns "sylvatic" plague, or plague occurring exclusively among wild rodents, such as prairie dogs in the western United States. With regard to "murine" plague, or plague occurring among domestic rat colonies living in people's homes, the Indian Plague Research Commission found that plague spread at a rate of 300 feet in six weeks, which is equivalent to about 2,600 feet in a year. See Indian Plague Research Commission, Reports on Plague Investigations in India, XXIII: "Epidemiological Observations in the Villages of Sion, Wadhala, Parel and Worli in Bombay Villages," *Journal of Hygiene* 7 (1907): 839.

[34]For example, Graham Twigg calculated that the Black Death, having arrived in Marseilles at the end of December 1347, traveled immediately due north overland to Paris, where it arrived at the end of June 1348, covering a distance of about 482 miles in 182 days, or at a rate of 2.5 miles per day. But an equally plausible scenario is that the Black Death came to Paris from the *north*, namely, from Rouen just inland from the Normandy coast, where it probably arrived by ship at the beginning of May 1348. This would mean that the Black Death traveled the 75 miles from Rouen to Paris in about 50 days, or at a rate of 1.5 miles per day, almost half the pace estimated by Twigg. See Twigg, *Black Death*, 139; Benedictow, *Black Death*, 107–8.

[35]Karl Sudhoff, "Pestschriften aus den ersten 150 Jahren nach der Epidemie des 'schwarzen Todes von 1348,'" *Archiv für Geschichte der Medizin (AGM)* 11 (1919): 47; Henricus de Hervordia, *Liber de Rebus Memorabilioribus sive Chronicon*, ed. Augustus Potthast (Göttingen, 1859), 280.

[36]Anne Karin Hufthammer and Lars Walløe, "Rats Cannot Have Been Intermediate Hosts for *Yersinia pestis* during Medieval Plague Epidemics in Northern Europe," *Journal of Archaeological Science* 40 (2013): 1753–56; Gunnar Karlsson, "Plague without Rats: The Case of Fifteenth-Century Iceland," *Journal of Medieval History* 22 (1996): 263–65, 276–80; David E. Davis, "The Scarcity of Rats and the Black Death: An Ecological History," *Journal of Interdisciplinary History* 16 (1986): 455–70; Cohn, *Black Death Transformed*, 1, 21–22, 81–82, 134; Twigg, *Black Death*, 111–12; Shrewsbury, *Bubonic Plague*, 7, 23, 53; Scott and Duncan, *Biology of Plagues*, 56–57.

[37]Michael McCormick, "Rats, Communications, and Plague: Toward an Ecological History," *Journal of Interdisciplinary History* 34 (2003): 5–6, 14; Anton Ervynk, "Sedentism or Urbanism? On the Origin of the Commensal Black Rat (*Rattus rattus*)," in *Bones and the Man: Studies in Honour of Don Brothwell*, ed. K. Dobney and T. O'Connor (Oxford: Oxbow Press, 2002), 95–96. McCormick states that the latest data on medieval rat archaeological finds "challenge the opinion that late medieval Europe had too few rats to have sustained bubonic plague during the Black Death." In fact, the most numerous rat finds have been found on sites dating to the thirteenth century or later, hinting at "hugely expanding rat populations" on the eve of the Black Death.

[38]McCormick, "Rats, Communications, and Plague," 4; Benedictow, *What Disease Was Plague?*, 134; Benedictow, *Black Death*, 24.

[39]Avicenna, *Liber Canonis* (Hildesheim: Georg Olms, 1964), fol. 416v. This testimony is mentioned by Cohn, who takes it as evidence that no one observed rat epizootics in the Middle Ages since all these animals were seen as issuing from their holes alive and were even captured alive. See Cohn, *Black Death Transformed*, 22, 133–34; Cohn, "Epidemiology of the Black Death," 78.

[40]Universitäts- und Forschungsbibliothek Gotha, Codex Chart. A 501, fols. 279r.-v.; Sudhoff, "Pestschriften," *AGM* 16 (1924–1925): 25. Saxony's testimony is mentioned by Cohn, but, once again, Cohn discounts it on the grounds that there is "no description of an epizootic of rodents; the mice were still alive." See Cohn, *Black Death Transformed*, 134.

[41]W. B. Bannerman, "The Spread of Plague in India," *Journal of Hygiene* 6 (1906): 183–84; Indian Plague Research Commission, Reports on Plague Investigations in India, XXXVI: "Observations of Plague in Belgaum, 1908–1909," *Journal of Hygiene* 10 (1910):

453–54; Indian Plague Research Commission, "Epidemiological Observations," 825, 836, 839, 845–46, 854, 869; Benedictow, *What Disease Was Plague?*, 92–97; L. Fabian Hirst, *The Conquest of Plague: A Study of the Evolution of Epidemiology* (Oxford: Clarendon Press, 1953), 147–48.

[42]Cohn, "Epidemiology of the Black Death," 76, 11n, 98; Cohn, "Historian and the Laboratory," 208.

[43]Cohn, *Black Death Transformed*, 77–78; Benedictow, *What Disease Was Plague?*, 340–80.

[44]Cohn, *Black Death Transformed*, 61–62.

[45]Sudhoff, "Pestschriften," *AGM* 11 (1919): 151.

[46]Benedictow, *What Disease Was Plague?*, 79–80, 346.

[47]Sudhoff, "Pestschriften," *AGM* 17 (1925): 113, 116.

[48]John Clynn, *Annalium Hiberniae Chronicon* (*The Annals of Ireland*), ed. Richard Butler (Dublin: Irish Archaeological Society, 1849), 37.

[49]Timothy Kircher, "Anxiety and Freedom in Boccaccio's History of the Plague of 1348," *Letteratura Italiana antica* 3 (2002): 319–57.

PART TWO

The Documents

1

Geographical Origins

Most chroniclers, whether Christian or Muslim, testify that the Black Death began somewhere in the East. Perhaps the most qualified commentator on plague's geographical origins is Abū Hafs ʿUmar Ibn al-Wardī (Document 2), who was based in Aleppo in northern Palestine and who gathered reports about the Black Death from Muslim merchants returning from Crimea, the westernmost terminus of the Mongol trade route across the Central Asian plateau.[1] Al-Wardī's preferred place of origin for the plague is the so-called land of darkness, perhaps referring to Mongolia, or "Inner Asia."[2] Christian authors, like Giovanni Villani (Document 3), were more concerned about describing plague's eastern origins in biblical terms, as a series of apocalyptic disasters, which nonetheless did not rule out more naturalistic explanations for the Black Death.[3] Genetic mapping of global samples of modern isolates of *Yersinia pestis* has allowed researchers to trace the earliest origins of plague to the Tibetan Plateau in China.[4] Around 1268, a "big bang" mutation occurred, when *Yersinia pestis* split into four other branches that are geographically plotted along the Silk Road in western China and Kurdistan.[5] This suggests that the disease traveled with goods on trade routes from one rat colony to another and that the particular strain or strains that caused the Black Death originated somewhere in Central Asia. Nonetheless, some object that plague could not have spread over such long distances in caravans transporting luxury goods through arid, desert-like climates, all of which would have been inhospitable to rats and fleas.[6] But travelers along the Silk Road typically moved in small circuits, or chains, from one oasis town to the next, often serving local markets with a variety of goods.[7] Moreover, the suggested alternative origin—in the Caucasus region of southern Russia—implies that plague reached no further east than Europe and never predated 1346–1347, which would go against most contemporary chronicles of the Black Death.[8]

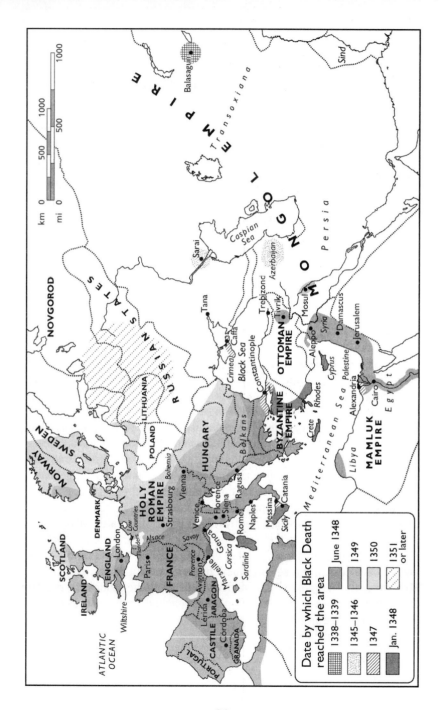

Date by which Black Death reached the area

1338–1339

1345–1346

1347

Jan. 1348

June 1348

1349

1350

1351 or later

MONGOL EMPIRE

Balasagun

Transoxiana

Sind

Persia

Caspian Sea

Azerbaijan

Sarai

Tana

Trebizond

Tivrik

Mosul

Caffa

Crimea

Black Sea

Constantinople

Aleppo

Syria

Damascus

Jerusalem

Palestine

Cyprus

Rhodes

OTTOMAN EMPIRE

BYZANTINE EMPIRE

Crete

Alexandria

Cairo

Egypt

Libya

MAMLUK EMPIRE

Mediterranean Sea

NOVGOROD

RUSSIAN STATES

LITHUANIA

POLAND

HUNGARY

Balkans

Ragusa

Vienna

Bohemia

HOLY ROMAN EMPIRE

Strasbourg

Venice

Florence

Siena

Rome

Naples

Messina

Catania

Sicily

Sardinia

Corsica

Genoa

Marseille

Savoy

Provence

Alsace

Low Countries

Flanders

London

Paris

FRANCE

Avignon

Roussillon

ARAGON

Lérida

CASTILE

Córdoba

GRANADA

PORTUGAL

ENGLAND

Wiltshire

SCOTLAND

IRELAND

NORWAY

SWEDEN

DENMARK

ATLANTIC OCEAN

km 0   500   1000
mi 0   500   1000

NOTES

[1] Michael W. Dols, *The Black Death in the Middle East* (Princeton, N.J.: Princeton University Press, 1977), 50–51.

[2] Ibid., 40, 49–50. Al-Wardī's account of the geographical origins of the Black Death is further strengthened by the discovery, in 1885, of three Nestorian headstones, listing ten people as dying of "pestilence" in 1338–1339, at Lake Issyk Kul in Kyrgyzstan, which lies along the overland route from Mongolia to Crimea. See John Norris, "East or West? The Geographic Origin of the Black Death," *Bulletin of the History of Medicine* 51 (1977): 10; Ole J. Benedictow, *The Black Death, 1346–1353: The Complete History* (Woodbridge, Suffolk: Boydell Press, 2004), 48.

[3] Laura A. Smoller, "Plague and the Investigation of the Apocalypse," in *Last Things: Death and the Apocalypse in the Middle Ages*, ed. Caroline Walker Bynum and Paul Freedman (Philadelphia: University of Pennsylvania Press, 2000), 156–88.

[4] The genetic focus of plague in the Tibetan Plateau (the "Microtus biovar") is closely related to other foci in Central Asia, including Mongolia, the Altaic region between Mongolia and Kazakhstan, and Tajikistan on the western border of China, as well as in the Caucasus. See Yanquin Li et al., "Genotyping and Phylogenetic Analysis of *Yersinia pestis* by MLVA: Insights into the Worldwide Expansion of Central Asia Plague Foci," *PLoS One* 4 (2009): online, e6000.

[5] Yujun Cui et al., "Historical Variations in Mutation Rate in an Epidemic Pathogen, *Yersinia pestis*," *Proceedings of the National Academy of Sciences* 110 (2013): 578–79; Giovanna Morelli et al., "Phylogenetic Diversity and Historical Patterns of Pandemic Spread of *Yersinia pestis*," *National Genetics* 42 (2010): 1141–42. Cui and his colleagues conclude, however, that this "big bang" mutation event around 1268 did not lead to greater virulence or a major new ability of *Yersinia pestis* to cause plague in humans, contrary to previous assumptions. See Kirsten I. Bos et al., "A Draft Genome of *Yersinia pestis* from Victims of the Black Death," *Nature* 478 (2011): 509.

[6] Ole J. Benedictow, "*Yersinia pestis*, the Bacterium of Plague, Arose in East Asia: Did It Spread Westwards via the Silk Roads, the Chinese Maritime Expeditions of Zheng He or over the Vast Eurasian Populations of Sylvatic (Wild) Rodents?," *Journal of Asian History* 47 (2013): 1–31; Benedictow, *Black Death*, 47–48; Norris, "East or West?," 15–16.

[7] Valerie Hansen, *The Silk Road: A New History* (Oxford: Oxford University Press, 2012), 5–10.

[8] Benedictow, *Black Death*, 49–51, and map 1; Norris, "East or West?," 11–24.

Opposite: The Path of the Black Death from Central Asia to Europe.

1

NICEPHORUS GREGORAS

Byzantine History

ca. 1359

An eminent historian and scholar writing in Constantinople, Nicephorus Gregoras provides important testimony to the arrival of plague in the Greek world. As court librarian to Emperor Andronikos III (1328–1341), Gregoras undoubtedly had access to some of the best records and sources then available. As the gateway to Crimea, Constantinople may have played a pivotal role in transmitting plague to the rest of the Mediterranean basin further south and west. This excerpt is from Gregoras's Historia Byzantina, *or* Byzantine History, *which covers the years 1204 to 1359. Gregoras died in 1360.*

During that time [1347], a serious and pestilential disease invaded humanity. Starting from Scythia [southern Russia] and Maeotis and the mouth of the Tanais [Don River], just as spring began, it lasted for that whole year, passing through and destroying, to be exact, only the continental coast, towns as well as country areas, ours and those that are adjacent to ours, up to Gadera and the columns of Hercules [Straits of Gibraltar].

During the second year [1348] it invaded the Aegean Islands. Then it affected the Rhodians, as well as the Cypriots and those colonizing the other islands. The calamity attacked men as well as women, rich and poor, old and young. To put matters simply, it did not spare those of any age or fortune. Several homes were emptied of all their inhabitants in one day or sometimes in two. No one could help anyone else, not even the neighbors, or the family, or blood relations.

The calamity did not destroy men only, but many animals living with and domesticated by men. I speak of dogs and horses and all the species of birds, even the rats that happened to live within the walls of

Christos S. Bartsocas, "Two Fourteenth-Century Greek Descriptions of the 'Black Death,'" *Journal of the History of Medicine and Allied Sciences* 21 (1966): 395. Reprinted by permission of Oxford University Press via Copyright Clearance Center.

the houses. The prominent signs of this disease, signs indicating early death, were tumorous outgrowths at the roots of thighs and arms and simultaneously bleeding ulcerations, which, sometimes the same day, carried the infected rapidly out of this present life, sitting or walking.

2

ABŪ HAFS ʿUMAR IBN AL-WARDĪ

Essay on the Report of the Pestilence

ca. 1348

Abū Hafs ʿUmar Ibn al-Wardī was born in northern Palestine between 1290 and 1292. After studying at Muslim schools in Syria, he served as deputy to the qadi, *or religious judge, of Aleppo until 1343, and thereafter devoted himself to writing. His collected works cover a range of topics, including grammar, history, law, mysticism, and the interpretation of dreams. Although plague came to Palestine in May or June 1348, it was not until March 18, 1349, that al-Wardī succumbed to the disease in Aleppo, near his birthplace. His* Risālah al-naba' ʿan al-waba' *(Essay on the Report of the Pestilence) was therefore written at the height of the epidemic. In addition, al-Wardī was in an ideal geographical position to comment on the plague's transmission from east to west. Scholars think that, like Gabriele de Mussis (Document 28), he benefited from plague reports he received from his mercantile colleagues. Using a style typical of Arabic scholastic writing, al-Wardī inserts poetic verses into the narrative to aid in memorization of the text.*

God is my security in every adversity. My sufficiency is in God alone. Is not God sufficient protection for His servant? Oh God, pray for our master, Muhammad, and give him peace. Save us for his sake from the attacks of the plague and give us shelter.

Michael W. Dols, "Ibn al-Wardī's *Risālah al-naba' ʿan al-waba'*, a Translation of a Major Source for the History of the Black Death in the Middle East," *Near Eastern Numismatics, Iconography, Epigraphy and History: Studies in Honor of George C. Miles,* ed. Dickran K. Kouymjian (Beirut: American University of Beirut, 1974), 447–51. Reprinted by permission of American University of Beirut.

The plague frightened and killed. It began in the land of darkness. Oh, what a visitor! It has been current for fifteen years. China was not preserved from it nor could the strongest fortress hinder it. The plague afflicted the Indians in India. It weighed upon the Sind.[1] It seized with its hand and ensnared even the lands of the Uzbeks. How many backs did it break in what is Transoxiana! The plague increased and spread further. It attacked the Persians, extended its steps toward the land of the Khitai,[2] and gnawed away at the Crimea. It pelted Rūm[3] with live coals and led the outrage to Cyprus and the islands. The plague destroyed mankind in Cairo. Its eye was cast upon Egypt, and behold, the people were wide-awake. It stilled all movement in Alexandria. The plague did its work like a silkworm. It took from the tiraz[4] factory its beauty and did to its workers what fate decreed.

Oh Alexandria, this plague is like a lion which extends its arm to you. Have patience with the fate of thc plague, which leaves of seventy men only seven.

Then, the plague turned to Upper Egypt. It, also, sent forth its storm to Barqa.[5] The plague attacked Gaza, and it shook Ascalon[6] severely. The plague oppressed Acre. The scourge came to Jerusalem and paid the zakat[7] [with the souls of men]. It overtook those people who fled to the al-ʿAqsā Mosque, which stands beside the Dome of the Rock.[8] If the door of mercy had not been opened, the end of the world would have occurred in a moment. It, then, hastened its pace and attacked the entire maritime plain. The plague trapped Sidon and descended unexpectedly upon Beirut, cunningly. Next, it directed the shooting of its arrows to Damascus. There the plague sat like a king on a throne and swayed with power, killing daily one thousand or more and decimating the population. It destroyed mankind with its pustules. May God the Most High spare Damascus to pursue its own path and extinguish the plague's fires so that they do not come close to her fragrant orchards. . . . The plague

---

[1]The region of the lower Indus river, along the present-day border between northwest India and Pakistan.

[2]Thought to be northeastern China (Khitai is Cathay, the medieval term for China), or the Jagatai Khanate of Turkestan.

[3]The Turkish realm of Anatolia, or modern-day Turkey.

[4]Tiraz refers to the silk and cloth manufacturing industry in Egypt.

[5]A province in present-day Libya.

[6]Both Gaza and Ascalon were important cities in southwestern Palestine.

[7]A tax on Muslims.

[8]The two most holy Muslim sites in Jerusalem.

domesticated itself in Hamā,[9] and the banks of the rivers ʿAsi became cold because of the plague's fever.

Oh Plague, Hamā is one of the best lands, one of the mightiest fortresses. Would that you had not breathed her air and poisoned her, kissing her and holding her in your embrace.

The plague entered Maʿarrat al-Nuʿmān and said to the city: "You are safe from me. Hamā is sufficient for your torture. I am satisfied with that."

It saw the town of Maʿarrat, like an eye adorned with blackness, but its eyebrow decorated with oppression.
What could the plague do in a country where every day its tyranny is a plague?

The plague and its poison spread to Sarmin.[10] It reviled the Sunni and the Shi'i.[11] It sharpened its spearheads for the Sunni and advanced like an army. The plague was spread in the land of the Shi'i with a ruinous effect. To Antioch the plague gave its share. Then, it left there quickly with a shyness like a man who has forgotten the memory of his beloved. Next, it said to Shayzar and to al-Hārim,[12] "Do not fear me. Before I come and after I go, you can easily disregard me because of your wretchedness. And the ruined places will recover from the time of the plague." Afterward, the plague humbled ʿAzaz and took from the people of al-Bāb[13] their men of learning. . . . Then, the plague sought Aleppo, but it did not succeed. By God's mercy the plague was the lightest oppression. I would not say that plants must grow from their seeds.

The pestilence had triumphed and appeared in Aleppo.
They said: It has made on mankind an attack. I called it a pestilence.

How amazingly does it pursue the people of each house! One of them spits blood, and everyone in the household is certain of death. It brings the entire family to their graves after two or three nights.

---

[9]A town about forty miles south of al-Wardī's birthplace of Maʿarrat.
[10]A town in northern Syria about midway between Antioch and Maʿarrat.
[11]Followers of two rival sects of Islam.
[12]Both in northern Syria about forty to fifty miles from Aleppo.
[13]Both towns are about twenty to twenty-six miles from Aleppo.

3

GIOVANNI VILLANI

Chronicle

ca. 1348

The son of a prosperous merchant, Giovanni Villani was one of the leading citizens of Florence in the early 1300s. He was a partner in two important banking houses and held the highest office in the Florentine Republic, the priorate, three times. At the age of twenty, during a pilgrimage to Rome, Villani was inspired to write a history of Florence, in imitation of ancient Latin authors. His Chronicle *is invaluable not only as a historical record but also as an important contribution to the vernacular literature being created by fellow Florentines, Dante, Petrarch (Document 11), and Boccaccio (Document 12). Villani died during the Black Death in 1348, while writing the latest installment to his history.*

This same pestilence was greater in Pistoia and Prato[1] than even in Florence with its high death rate. Still greater were the deaths in Bologna and the Romagna and worse at the papal court in Avignon in Provence, and in all of the kingdom of France. But there were uncountable deaths in Turkey and other countries overseas, where the disease lasted longer and did the most harm. God's justice fell harshly among the Tartars [Mongols], so much so that it seemed incredible. It is true, clear, and certain that in the land between the Turks and Chinese, in the country of Parthia, now named the Khanate [of the Mongols, or the Ilkhan Empire], the leader of the Tartars in India began a fire that shot out from the ground. In other words, this flame would come down from the sky and destroy men, animals, houses, trees, rocks and the land. This distended fire burned for more than fifteen days and became quite troublesome. He who did not flee fell victim to its wrath, and it continuously burned every animal and person. The men and women who managed to escape the fires would die of the plague. In Tana [Azov] and

[1] Two other towns in Tuscany near Florence.

Giovanni Villani, *Nuova cronica*, ed. Giuseppe Porta, 3 vols. (Parma: Fondazione Pietro Bembo, 1990–1991), 3:486–88. Translated from the Italian by Aubrey Threlkeld.

Trebizond, and in all of the surrounding territories, few remained and the number lost was as high as five men for every one survivor. Most of the land was uninhabited due to the plagues, as well as to the enormous earthquakes and lightning. And according to some letters from trustworthy citizens of our town who were in the area, such as at Sivas [in Anatolia], it rained an immeasurable quantity of vermin,[2] some as big as eight hands, all black and with tails, some alive and some dead. This frightening scene was made worse by the stench that they emitted, and those who fought against the vermin fell victim to their venom. And in another countryside, in Greece, no one remained alive unless they were female, and even some of them died because of rabies. And a more amazing and almost incredible event came to pass in Arcadia:[3] Men and women and every living animal turned into the likeness of marble statues. The mayors from the surrounding areas stated that this must be a sign to convert to the Christian faith; but they heard from news on the western wind that even Christian lands were troubled with pestilence, so they continued to practice their own religious treachery [Islam].[4] In the port of Talucco, in [the contado or district of] Lucca, the sea was filled with vermin, better than 10,000 between the seas. Leaving them there, they [Muslims] went from one place to another until they arrived at Lucca, where out of their strong admiration for Christianity, they immediately converted. These pestilences occurred as far away as Turkey and Greece, having come from the area of the rising sun in Mesopotamia, Syria, Chaldea, Cyprus, the islands of Crete and Rhodes, and all of the islands in the Greek Archipelago. And then it happened in Sicily, Sardinia, Corsica, and Elba, and in a similar way on the coastlines and in the rivers of our seas. And of eight Genoese galleys that were stationed in the Black Sea, where many died, only four of them returned, full of the sick and dying. And all those who reached Genoa were nearly dead, and upon their arrival they corrupted the air that they breathed, so much so that whoever offered them refuge would soon die. . . . And this pestilence lasted until _____,[5] and many areas of the city and in the provinces remained desolate.

---

[2]Villani seems to refer here to black rats, which we know from modern experience to be vectors of bubonic plague. It is even possible that rats did "rain" from the ceilings of houses, as they fell down dead from the disease.

[3]A territory in Greece on the Peloponnesus, just north of the ancient kingdom of Sparta.

[4]A similar tale is told by several other chroniclers.

[5]Here the chronicle is simply left blank.

2

Symptoms and Transmission

The way that medieval people conceived of plague—including its symptoms and how it was transmitted from one person, region, or community to another—is largely foreign to our modern approach to disease. And yet, some medieval medical theories—such as that the groin, armpits, and neck served as "emunctories," or drainage points, for plague matter—are remarkably prescient. Nonetheless, as mentioned in the introduction, some scholars believe that there is an "unbridgeable gap" between the premodern concept of plague and the modern, "laboratory construction" of the disease—that is, one based on the identification of microorganisms in infected victims.[1] In addition, premodern descriptions of symptoms—even when provided by medieval doctors—should, in this view, never be compared with modern diagnoses, since the respective concepts of disease are just too different.[2] But paleomicrobiology has now demonstrated that the techniques of the laboratory can be made to successfully isolate *Yersinia pestis* in victims of the Black Death, proving that premodern and modern versions of plague are, indeed, one and the same.[3] This means, in turn, "that it is not possible to reject the plague etiology of the Black Death simply because certain symptoms and epidemiological features do not match those found today."[4]

Instead, one must carefully consider the context of each contemporary description of the Black Death in order to determine its reliability and value. This is especially the case with the more literary accounts of plague, such as those by Louis Sanctus (Document 4) and John VI Kantakouzenos (Document 5). For some historians, the main goal of the medieval chronicler was not to provide an eyewitness account of the Black Death but, rather, "to serve his (legitimate) literary purpose of dramatization."[5] In this view, medieval authors had a "much weaker empirical orientation" than their modern counterparts, and their writings about plague must be judged accordingly.[6] This would apply even to more scientific works, such as the plague treatises written by medieval physicians. However, the treatise by the Moorish doctor Abū Ja'far Ahmad Ibn Khātima (Document 6) is rather unique in that it showcases Khātima's own empirical observation (including case histories of patients) to describe the symptoms of the Black Death. Indeed, Khātima provides almost a textbook clinical diagnosis of the three forms of plague: bubonic, pneumonic, and septicemic. But Khātima also describes things that, from a modern perspective, we know to be untrue, such as that plague was transmitted via miasmas, or infected vapors in the air. Nonetheless, even here, his account is still valuable for the window it provides onto the mind-set and views of his contemporaries with respect to disease.

NOTES

[1]Andrew Cunningham, "Transforming Plague: The Laboratory and the Identity of Infectious Disease," in *The Laboratory Revolution in Medicine*, ed. Andrew Cunningham and Perry Williams (Cambridge: Cambridge University Press, 1992), 242.

[2]Ibid., 242 and 47*n*. Indeed, Cunningham ridicules any attempt to identify past diseases in this manner as "bizarre."

[3]Ibid., 216.

[4]Elizabeth Carniel, "Plague Today," in *Pestilential Complexities: Understanding Medieval Plague*, ed. Vivian Nutton (*Medical History*, Supplement no. 27, 2008), 122.

[5]Ole J. Benedictow, *What Disease Was Plague? On the Controversy over the Microbiological Identity of Plague Epidemics of the Past* (Leiden: Brill, 2010), 361.

[6]Ibid., 79–80, 346.

4

LOUIS SANCTUS

Letter

April 27, 1348

In the following excerpt from his letter of April 27, 1348, written from Avignon, Louis Sanctus describes three forms of the disease, although it is not clear that these necessarily correspond to bubonic, pneumonic, and septicemic plague. Because Avignon was at the time the seat of the papacy, expert medical attention was available in the city and, by Sanctus's account, autopsies were conducted on plague victims. Sanctus seems to have had access to such expert medical testimony when writing his description of the symptoms of the disease, particularly of the pneumonic variety.

Recueil des chroniques de Flandre, ed. Joseph-Jean de Smet, 4 vols. (Brussels, 1837–1865), 3:5–16.

And it is said that the plague is of three types of infection. First, that men feel pain in their lungs, from which there comes a shortness of breath. He who has this malady, or is contaminated by it in any way whatsoever, can in no way escape, but will not live more than two days. Indeed, dissections were carried out by doctors in many Italian cities, and also in Avignon by order and command of the pope, so that the origin of this plague might be known. And many dead bodies were cut up and opened, and it was found that all who die so suddenly have an infection of the lungs and spit up blood. And thus it follows that this plague is indeed most terrible and dangerous to all, namely that it is contagious, because whenever one infected person dies, all who see him during his illness, or visit him, or have dealings with him in any way, or carry him to his grave, straightaway follow him [to their deaths], without any remedy.

There is also another kind of plague, that at present exists alongside the aforesaid [pneumonic plague]: namely that certain apostemes [tumors] suddenly appear on both armpits, from which men die without delay. And there is even a third plague, likewise concurrent with the two mentioned above, but at present it runs its own course: namely that people of both sexes are stricken in the groin, from which they die suddenly. As the aforesaid plague spreads, it has come to pass that the doctor does not visit the sick for fear of this contagion, not even if the patient would give him everything he possessed in this life. Nor does the father visit his son, the mother her daughter, brother his brother, the son his father, the friend his friend, the acquaintance his acquaintance, nor anyone another who may be a blood relation, unless he wishes to suddenly die like him or follow him [to the grave] immediately. And thus an innumerable number of men have died who did their affectionate duty to their relations and who also were known for their piety and charity, but who perchance might have escaped had they not visited them at the time.

5

JOHN VI KANTAKOUZENOS

History

1367–1369

A member of the powerful Kantakouzenos family that owned large estates in Thrace, John VI became emperor of Byzantium in 1341 as the result of a coup in which he claimed to be acting as regent for the legitimate heir to the throne, John V Paleologus. But in 1354, John V, who had attained his majority, forced John VI to abdicate and retire to a monastery. Kantakouzenos used his retirement to write his History of the Byzantine Empire, *which he seems to have composed into its final form between 1367 and 1369. Although some scholars think that Kantakouzenos imitated the literary style of the ancient Greek historian Thucydides in this passage, his detailed observations on plague appear to be genuine. The plague of Athens of 430–426 BCE (now thought to be typhoid fever) was a different disease from the Black Death. The emperor had the opportunity to observe this firsthand when his youngest son, Andronikos, succumbed on the third day after plague struck Constantinople. John VI himself lived to 1383.*

So incurable was the evil, that neither any regularity of life, nor any bodily strength could resist it. Strong and weak bodies were all similarly carried away, and those best cared for died in the same manner as the poor. No other disease of any kind presented itself that year. If someone had a previous illness he always succumbed to this disease and no physician's art was sufficient; neither did the disease take the same course in all persons, but the others, unable to resist, died the same day, a few even within the hour. Those who could resist for two or three days had a very violent fever at first, the disease in such cases attacking the head; they suffered from speechlessness and insensibility to all happenings and then appeared as if sunken into a deep sleep. Then, if from time to

Christos S. Bartsocas, "Two Fourteenth-Century Greek Descriptions of the 'Black Death,'" *Journal of the History of Medicine and Allied Sciences* 21 (1966): 396. Reprinted by permission of Oxford University Press via Copyright Clearance Center.

time they came to themselves, they wanted to speak but the tongue was hard to move and they uttered inarticulate sounds because the nerves around the occiput [back of the head] were dead; and they died suddenly. In others, the evil attacked not the head, but the lung, and forthwith there was inflammation inside which produced very sharp pains in the chest.

Sputum suffused with blood was brought up and disgusting and stinking breath from within. The throat and tongue, parched from the heat, were black and congested with blood. It made no difference if they drank much or little. Sleeplessness and weakness were established forever.

Abscesses formed on the upper and lower arms, in a few also in the maxillae [jaw], and in others on other parts of the body. In some they were large and in others small. Black blisters appeared. Some people broke out with black spots all over their bodies; in some they were few and very manifest; in others they were obscure and dense. Everyone died the same death from these symptoms. In some people all the symptoms appeared, in others more or fewer of them, and in no small number even one of these was sufficient to provoke death. Those few who were able to escape from among the many who died were no longer possessed by the same evil, but were safe. The disease did not attack twice in order to kill them.

Great abscesses were formed on the legs or the arms, from which, when cut, a large quantity of foul-smelling pus flowed and the disease was differentiated as that which discharged much annoying matter. Even many who were seized by all the symptoms unexpectedly recovered. There was no help from anywhere; if someone brought to another a remedy useful to himself, this became poison to the other patient. Some, by treating others, became infected with the disease. . . . Most terrible was the discouragement. Whenever people felt sick there was no hope left for recovery, but by turning to despair, adding to their prostration and severely aggravating their sickness, they died at once. No words could express the nature of the disease.

6

ABŪ JA'FAR AHMAD IBN KHĀTIMA

Description and Remedy for Escaping the Plague

February 1349

A physician and poet from Almería on the coast of southern Spain, at that time part of the Muslim kingdom of Granada, Abū Ja'far Ahmad Ibn Khātima wrote his plague treatise in February 1349. Although grounding himself in earlier theory, such as that of Hippocrates, Galen, and Avenzoar (Ibn Zuhr), particularly with regard to explaining the causes of plague, Khātima also seems to speak from experience as the result of diagnosing and treating plague patients after the Black Death arrived in Almería on June 1, 1348. His treatise, titled Tahsīl al-gharad al-qāsid fī tafsīl al-marad al-wāfid *(A Description and Remedy for Escaping the Plague in the Future), is the most detailed of the few medical works in Arabic to have survived from the time of the Black Death. Khātima lived until at least 1369, when he is mentioned by his friend and fellow physician Lisān al-Dīn Ibn al-Khatīb (Document 21). The following selection is from the first, fourth, and sixth questions of Khātima's treatise.*

Particularities of the disease. . . . We say, then, with the help of God Almighty, that this [plague] is a malignant, continuous fever, coming from the morbidity of the internal temperament which is due to the degradation of the air, the same being caused by the evolution of its natural state into qualities of heat and moisture. The fever is very often deadly, accompanied by anxiety and localized sweats, which are not followed by feelings of calm nor by a rise in temperature. On the second day, one observes most of the time depression and disorientation. Then the fever climbs higher and is followed by: cramps; coldness in the extremities; frightful, bilious, recurring vomiting; diverse lesions on the skin; or: a tightness in the chest; difficulty in breathing; spitting of blood or stinging pain on the

Abū Ğa'far ibn Ḥātima al-Anṣārī, *La Grande Peste en Espagne Musulmane au XIVᵉ Siècle: Taḥṣīl garad al-qāṣid fī tafṣīl al-marad al-wāfid*, trans. and ed. Suzanne Gigandet (Damascus: Institut français du Proche-Orient, 2010), 20, 39–41, 53–54, 58–60, 68–69; Taha Dinānah, "Ibn Hātimah über die Pest: die Schrift von Abī Ğa'far Ahmed ibn 'Alī ibn Mohammed ibn 'Alī ibn Hātimah aus Almeriah," *Archiv für Geschichte der Medizin* 19 (1927): 32–33, 49–51, 59–60, 64–66, 77–78.

side or just below the breast, accompanied by inflammation and an intense thirst; coughing; blackness of tongue or swelling of the throat with complications of quinsy [i.e., a peritonsillar abscess]; and a difficulty or impossibility of swallowing; or: headaches; fainting fits; dizziness; nausea and foul-smelling diarrhea. Sometimes certain of these signs exist alongside each other; sometimes they are accompanied by swellings of the glands, by pestilential bubos on the armpits, on the groin, behind the ears, or on the neighboring regions, preceded or not with pain. Sometimes there are black boils in diverse places of the body, but particularly on the back or on the neck, and sometimes also on the extremities. . . .

Infection.   It is a fact that one cannot hide, nor ignore: the ravages of this disease spread and cross borders. Testimony and experience confirm that it will not be very long before a healthy individual, who lives in the vicinity of a sick man, surrounded by the sickness, is stricken to his core and afflicted with the same disease. This is a nearly absolute law that comes from the Most High God, for, in reality, the action of an illness that exerts itself upon the first and second individual is the manifestation of His greatness, He who is the creator of all things. In this way we reject the beliefs of those who are in error insofar as the generation [of illnesses], the beliefs that were held by the Arabs in the time of the *Jahiliyya.*[1] And this confirms the reality to which we bear witness. . . .

We say then—may God help us!—that the root cause of the disease is a change in the air and its change into a second nature that replaces its normal one. And there is no more serious alteration and corruption [of the air] than that caused by the miasmas that emanate from sick men afflicted by this epidemic, and most particularly those who breathe their last, when their bodies and their breath are completely putrefied as death approaches. No one can breathe in these harmful, putrid, poisonous emanations but that they act upon him and facilitate his contamination, according to the degree of his predisposition and susceptibility [to the disease]. . . .

In the same way that the disease spreads by breath, it can be spread by the miasmas that arise from diseased bodies, and likewise without that [miasma], the body can only exert a weak influence [upon others]. The sick carry their illness in their clothes and in their bedding, and

---

[1]*Jahiliyya* refers to the "days of ignorance" in Arabia prior to its conversion to Islam. Here Khātima is paying lip service to the prophetic tradition in Islam that "there is no infection" or contagion of disease. Obviously, this goes against Khātima's own observation and experience, as well as that of his colleagues, such as Lisān al-Dīn Ibn al-Khatīb (Document 21).

especially if these have been in contact with the bodies or if they have been breathed upon. These are facts confirmed by science [i.e., knowledge] and experience.

I have observed that among the merchants at the *Suk el Haik* [secondhand clothes market] in Almería, who sell the clothes and bedding of the dead, a [large] number of them die, [and] only a very small number survive, and such [is the case] up to the present time. But those who live in the districts of other *suks* [markets] suffer [from plague] in the common way like [all the other] inhabitants of the town.

I have been informed of the situation of countries where the inhabitants decided, in order that they might protect themselves, that no one could enter there if he came from a region where the plague was raging. They have been able to remain safe for a certain amount of time, but the disease ended up striking them down as well. Most of the occupants of the fortresses surrounding Almería date the arrival of the scourge among them with a person, man or woman, who came from an infected region and died in their midst. A lot of reports are circulating on the subject of their precautions; these come in periodically, and there is no reason to contest them.

What we learn from our extensive applied practice [of medicine] is, based on our observations and upon reflection, extraordinary: He who is in frequent contact with a sick man stricken by this epidemic becomes himself the victim of an identical illness and presents the same symptoms. If the first man vomits blood, the other one does too. If one suffers from quinsy, the other suffers from this equally. If the inguinal glands swell up on one, it is the same for the other. If ulcers [boils] appear on the body of one, they afflict the other also. He who lives in close proximity to a sick man becomes his likeness, to the point that those who dwell in the same house [with the second man] are all stricken by the same kind of disease and by identical manifestations. If the first sick man dies, the others share his fate, and if he recovers, the others are safe also. This was how the epidemic progressed among the population of our country in the majority of cases. One can have exceptions, but what we describe is nearly always the rule. . . .

Treatment of the disease once it appears, but before it is established and worsens [in the body]. Know that these epidemic fevers are different from other fevers and can present contrary aspects. The usual fevers are classified into four categories. . . . [These are listed as: (1) fevers caused by corruption of the humors, mainly blood, yellow bile, and phlegm; (2) fevers caused by overheating of the vegetable, animal, and intellectual spirits; (3) fevers caused by heat and moisture in the bodily constitution and essential organs; (4) fevers that accompany illness.]

The epidemic fever of the present day differs in all respects from the preceding fevers. In the first place, its heat fixes itself in the heart and corrupts the heart's constitution and blood. But the progress of the disease is opposite to that of the other fevers, its evolution is different, and it doesn't proceed in stages. [Instead] the body suffers from disparate, strange symptoms and from abnormal conditions, similar to how a disorganized town appears, because the heart [which is under attack] governs the whole of the body and protects it. . . .

Treatments once the disease triumphs and is established [in the body]. . . . We say then that at the beginning of this kind of disease . . . the expulsive force that is within [the patient], along with what little energy has been husbanded, drives the corrupt part of the blood to the nearest places that are most apt for collecting it. If the body remains robust, healthy, and free of corrupt humors [and] if the portion of afflicted blood is only moderately irksome and unnatural, then this expulsive force should drive it towards the places of the body that naturally collect the superfluities, namely, behind the ears, on the armpits and on the groin, depending on the fluidity, density, thickness, and other relevant qualities [of the corrupt blood]. If the superfluity is thin and irksome, it is localized in the upper part of the body, and the brain drives it to behind the ears, the place most apt to receive it. If the superfluity is thick and heavy, it descends towards the lower part [of the body], and the liver drives it to the groin, which is the nearest place to receive the expelled materials of the liver. If the superfluity is midway between being thick and being runny, it is expelled to the armpits, which receive the superfluities of the heart. These are the places where glandular swellings form underneath the skin, which are hard [and] bloody, where the superfluities have collected. These are the pestiferous bubos, whose size and number [on the body] vary. And their quantity depends on the degree to which the superfluities have won over the neighboring regions, where they appear as new glandular swellings, which [in turn] depends on the aptitude [of these regions] for receiving them and that of the vessels through which they circulate.

If the [body's] expulsive force directs the superfluities towards an internal organ that is weak and vulnerable—in this case, the lungs—it is not long, or maybe it is a little while later, before the sick man suddenly spits up blood. This is caused by the caustic nature of the humor and by the impotence and weakness of the [lung] vessels. The lung, being a soft organ, is incapable of vanquishing this [expulsive] force and of resisting the driving pressure of the unnatural humor. Such is most often the case, but it also happens, albeit rarely, that it produces pneumonia. In cases where the liver is predisposed to and receives the humor, then this causes an inflamed tumor: When this is driven towards the diaphragm, pleurisy ensues; towards the intercostal muscles [of the ribs], then there is a sharp pleurisy [i.e., a stabbing pain]; towards the throat, then there is difficulty swallowing [from soreness or swelling]; towards the brain, then a *sirsām* or phrenitis, an acute inflammation [of the brain—i.e., frenzy] ensues and an intense fever. Sometimes two organs are afflicted at once by the abundance of this humor, and they are both predisposed to retain it.

If the expulsive forces have not encountered a weak internal organ, and if the humor is very caustic, they direct it to the surface of the body, where it develops into repulsive black ulcers, especially on the back, on the neck, and more rarely, on the extremities, depending on the predisposition of the spot to it. But God is the most wise!

Among the diverse forms of the plague, the three most common in man are the bubonic and blood-spitting forms and the one where black ulcers are formed.

If you ask why these three forms, and no others, are the most common, I answer:

The pestiferous bubos. This has entirely to do with receptivity. The bubos form on the places of the body designed by nature to receive the superfluities coming from the noble organs. God, in his divine wisdom, ordained that the noble organs, in order that they be protected against danger, drive the superfluities back towards the "inferior" zones [i.e., behind the ears, the armpits, or the groin], which are more ready to receive the superfluities than the noble organs, which are less disposed to collect them. Generally, then, our first care is to sacrifice these creases [glands] in the body to the benefit of the vital organs. These organs expel their superfluities through vessels that end up at the creases, where they find the glandular tissues and the slack is ready to take up the residue. And the cavities in the tissues expand, performing a function like the gutters in front of houses, into which one throws sweepings and refuse that the dwelling must disgorge, being unable to support them any longer. Glory be to God, who is goodness and light!

The blood-spitting form. This is caused by the proximity of the heart to the lungs, whose loose tissues and expansive cavities dispose them to receive the superfluities. Moreover, one's natural constitution is eager to expel this virulent residue from the heart, which cannot endure it, to the nearest place by means of an expulsive action.

The black ulcers.   An expulsive force acts to drive the residues towards the exterior of the body. The internal organs are in this way relieved by a force protecting them from their lack of receptivity to this very bitter and burning humor. This humor is directed towards the surface and goes out to the exterior [of the body]; it is not localized in the creases by reason of the rapidity and force of its expulsion. It is in this way that these ulcers are formed, by a process different from that for the other forms of the disease. God is the most wise!

The corruption of the heart's temperament [that is behind the black ulcers] may be due to an internal cause, such as bad nourishment or disturbed sleep, [or] it may be due to an external one, such as breathing in of unhealthy vapors, or [it may be due to] exposure to poisons and, generally speaking, to anything that destroys the natural defenses [of the body] and that renders [the body's] natural constitution impotent in the face of a weakening of [the body's] innate heat and expulsive force. Such is the case for a disease that kills suddenly, without showing the symptoms of one of the forms of the plague that we have described. . . .

The first form [of plague], that of pestiferous bubos.   These can be diagnosed by palpation or by the occurrence of a sharp pain or pressure in the stricken place [i.e., behind the ears, in the armpits, or in the groin]. But pain can be absent, for the symptoms of all forms of the disease are the same, or are very close to each other, in the beginning. Very often one observes shiverings, pain in the bones and a heaviness in the members, spasms in the blood vessels, [and] a gentle heat given off by the body, but perchance contrary signs are observed. . . . Urine is normal or nearly clear on the first day; then on the second or third day, it is purple, then of various colors. This is the general prognosis, but it can go the opposite way, depending on the temperaments [of patients]. As for pulse, in the beginning of the disease, it is agitated, racing; then, at the end, it becomes disordered. The [patient's] agitation is intense in general, but the diseased state is very variable: It cannot be soothed, and one should not rely on an appearance of health, for the symptoms of infection can resemble those of health. . . .

The second form [of the disease] is blood-spitting. . . .   It appears to me that all those who suffer from blood-spitting have no other reliable signs, neither pain nor fever, none of whom survive to the next day. And in particular, those who have been in contact with a deceased victim are exposed to very great danger. . . . Very often the blood brought up is black, for the blood from the lungs is dead, due to the fact that the innate heat is extinguished. Finally, the blood is completely corrupted, although the sick man feels no pain, the substance of the lungs being nearly insensible. Nonetheless, the sick man sometimes feels a pain in his side or under the breast, which is symptomatic and due to the compression of the diaphragm and to the propulsion of this [diseased] matter to the intercostal muscles [i.e., the muscles between the ribs]. God is the most wise, glory to Him!

The third form is that of the black ulcers.   These at first have the appearance of blackish swellings that [then] turn red as if from the action of the body's burning heat, and this is accompanied by inflammation and heat [in the ulcers]. Then these swellings burst open from the action of a corrupt matter, and they give way to black spots from which exudes a liquid, and often they are surrounded by an inflamed area. This is the most frequent diagnosis, but sometimes the spots appear at first to be distinct and resemble black grain kernels, or they turn red and swell out. Then they ulcerate when the matter that is shut up inside them becomes irritated. And while the glandular swellings of the groin and the armpits may have an excessive heat, the inflammation of the surrounding area [of the black ulcers] is extreme and causes pricking sensations, they ripen and exude their contents. And the sick man is [now] generally out of danger, for the adjoining flesh is consolidated, dried out, particularly in the case of bodies with a dry temperament. One can then remove them by cutting them out, for they are flush [with the skin], like the dried-out glandular swellings, which do not adhere [to the skin] and from which a watery humor flows out. The healing is then complete, particularly for ulcers on the creases of the body.

3

Medical Responses

Misconceptions about the medical response to the Black Death are legion. One of the most oft-repeated assertions is that medieval medicine remained stuck in the ancient rut of the humoral theory of disease, the principles of which go back to the ancient Greek physicians Hippocrates and Galen. This theory dictated that the body's complexion was composed of four humors—blood, phlegm, yellow bile, and black bile—which would cause illness when out of balance. There was thus little to no progress or change in medieval medicine, even in the face of a cataclysmic crisis on the order of the Black Death.[1]

There is evidence, however, that plague doctors did develop a new, alternative theory to explain the Black Death: the poison thesis (not to be confused with the poison conspiracy, discussed in Chapter 6). This was the idea that people became sick with plague because their bodies were invaded from the outside by a foreign substance, namely, by the worst kind of poison—one that acted through its "whole substance" or "specific form," which bypassed the humors and went straight to the heart, killing swiftly. Poison could also multiply itself once inside the body, converting "whatever it touches in the human body into [its own] poisonous form."[2] For a universal disease event like the Black Death, which seemed to afflict everyone indiscriminately, poison offered a universal cause that better fit the realities of plague's virulence than did humoral imbalance, which varied considerably from patient to patient. It seems that the Black Death epidemic was the first time that poison was conceptually applied to disease, in that those who were afflicted with plague were now believed to have been poisoned, whether naturally through the environment or artificially by human agency, namely through water, food, and even the air, according to Alfonso de Córdoba (Document 8).[3]

The Perugian physician Gentile da Foligno (Document 9) was the first to suggest poison as a natural cause of plague.[4] Poison implied a different treatment regimen for plague, one that relied more on drug therapies, such as theriac (an ancient cure for poison), and on sweating remedies (which aimed to heat up the body, something that was counterintuitive to humoral theory). Such ideas arguably laid the groundwork for the modern germ theory of disease (that is, that illness is caused by invading microorganisms, like bacteria) to emerge in the nineteenth century. At the same time, however, the poison thesis perhaps provided the logical underpinnings for the poison conspiracy to take hold in much of Europe during the Black Death, which tragically took the lives of thousands of Jews and other victims accused of intentionally spreading the plague by poisoning springs and wells (see Chapter 6).

NOTES

[1] Dominick Palazzotto, "The Black Death and Medicine: A Report and Analysis of the Tractates Written between 1348 and 1350" (Ph.D. diss., University of Kansas, 1973), 60–61; Norman F. Cantor, *In the Wake of the Plague: The Black Death and the World It Made* (New York: Free Press, 2001), 9; John Kelly, *The Great Mortality: An Intimate History of the Black Death, the Most Devastating Plague of All Time* (New York: HarperCollins, 2005), 163–75; Christiane Nockels Fabbri, "Continuity and Change in Late Medieval Plague Medicine: A Survey of 152 Plague Tracts from 1348 to 1599" (Ph.D diss., Yale University, 2006).

[2] Pietro d'Abano, *De Venenis* (Mantua: Johannes Vurster, 1473), fol. 8r; Melissa P. Chase, "Fevers, Poisons, and Apostemes: Authority and Experience in Montpellier Plague Treatises," *Annals of the New York Academy of Sciences* 441 (1985): 156–57.

[3] Chase, "Fevers, Poisons, and Apostemes," 155–56, 162; Frederick W. Gibbs, "Medical Understandings of Poison circa 1250–1600" (Ph.D. diss., University of Wisconsin–Madison, 2009), 106–7.

[4] Foligno, in turn, seems to have derived his ideas on poison from his teacher at the University of Padua, Pietro d'Abano, who wrote an influential treatise on poisons (the *De Venenis*) shortly before the onset of the Black Death. See Abano, *De Venenis*, fol. 3r.

7

MEDICAL FACULTY
OF THE UNIVERSITY OF PARIS

Consultation

October 6, 1348

On October 6, 1348, the college of the faculty of medicine at the University of Paris issued a compendium of opinion on the Black Death, apparently in response to a request from the king of France, Philip VI. In addition to relying on their own knowledge and ancient authorities like

H. Émile Rébouis, *Étude historique et critique sur la Peste* (Paris: A. Picard, 1888), 76–92.

Aristotle, the faculty members consulted "very many knowledgeable men in modern astrology and medicine concerning the causes of the epidemic which has been abroad since 1345." Their pronouncement therefore contained what was considered the most up-to-date scientific information available at the time and quickly became authoritative, as evidenced by its repetition in other plague treatises. The first part of the faculty's treatise addresses the "causes of this pestilence" and is divided into three chapters: one on a "distant" cause "which is up above and in the heavens," a second on a "near" cause "which is lower and on earth," and the third on "prognostications and signs, which are connected to both [above causes]." The second part, devoted to preventions and cures, is omitted because it covers much the same ground as Documents 9 and 10.

Concerning the Universal and Distant Cause. Therefore we say that the distant and first cause of this pestilence was and is a certain configuration in the heavens. In the year of our Lord 1345, at precisely one hour past noon on the twentieth day of the month of March,[1] there was a major conjunction [lining up] of three higher planets in Aquarius. Indeed, this conjunction, together with other prior conjunctions and eclipses, being the present cause of the ruinous corruption of the air that is all around us, is a harbinger of mortality and famine and many other things besides, which we will not touch on here because it does not pertain to our subject. Moreover, that this is so is testified by the philosopher, Aristotle, in his book, *Concerning the Causes of the Properties of the Elements.*[2] Around the middle [of the work] he says that mortalities of men and depopulation of kingdoms happen whenever there is a conjunction of two planets, namely Saturn and Jupiter, so that on account of their interaction disasters are magnified threefold to the third power [i.e., nine times], and all this is to be found in [the writings of] ancient philosophers. And Albertus [Magnus] says in his book, *Concerning the Causes of the Properties of the Elements*[3] (treatise 2, chapter 1), that a conjunction of two planets, namely Mars and Jupiter, brings about a great pestilence in the air, and

---

[1]The Paris masters most likely got this date from the *Prognosticatio* of Johannes de Muris, one of the astronomers summoned to the court of Pope Clement VI at Avignon in 1344–1345.

[2]This work was not by Aristotle but was commonly attributed to him. Aristotle was considered the leading authority of the ancient world and thus was invoked to support all kinds of positions.

[3]Albertus Magnus wrote commentaries on all of Aristotle's known works, which explains the similarity in the titles by the two authors.

that this happens especially under a hot and humid sign [i.e., Aquarius], as was the case when the planets lined up [in 1345]. For at that time, Jupiter, being hot and wet, drew up evil vapors from the earth, but Mars, since it is immoderately hot and dry, then ignited the risen vapors, and therefore there were many lightning flashes, sparks, and pestiferous vapors and fires throughout the atmosphere. . . .

Concerning the Particular and Near Cause. Although pestilential sicknesses can arise from a corruption of water and food, as happens in times of famine and poor productivity, nevertheless we are of the opinion that illnesses which proceed from a corruption of the air are more deadly, since this evil is more hurtful than food or drink in that its poison penetrates quickly to the heart and lungs. Moreover, we believe that the present epidemic or plague originated from air that was corrupt in its substance, and not only in its altered properties.[4] For we wish it to be understood that air, which is pure and clear by nature, does not putrefy or become corrupt unless it is mixed up with something else, that is, with evil vapors. For many vapors that had been corrupted at the time of the aforesaid conjunctions arose, by virtue of their [nature], from the earth and water, and in the air were spread and multiplied by frequent gusts of thick, wild, and southerly winds, which, on account of the foreign vapors they have brought and are still bringing with them, have corrupted the air in its substance. Thus, the corrupted air, when it is breathed in, necessarily penetrates to the heart and corrupts the substance of the spirit that is in it and putrefies the surrounding moisture, so that the heat that is created goes forth and by its nature corrupts the principle of life, and this is the immediate cause of the current epidemic. What is more, these winds, which have become so prevalent around us, could by their force have brought or carried to us, or perhaps will do so in the future, evil, putrid and poisonous vapors from afar, as, for instance, from swamps, lakes, deep valleys, and, in addition, from dead, unburied or unburned bodies, all of which are deadly. And this could be a cause of the epidemic. And possibly this corruption could have or will come

---

[4]The miasmatic theory of disease, that epidemics resulted from a substantial change in the quality of the air, was first advanced by Hippocratic writers and later championed by Galen. The Paris masters seem to define plague as a *result* of the substantial change in air, rather than as the change itself. Jacme d'Agramont (Document 10), an anonymous Montpellier practitioner, and Gentile da Foligno (Document 9) took an opposite view. For more on this debate, see Jon Arrizabalaga, "Facing the Black Death: Perceptions and Reactions of University Medical Practitioners," in *Practical Medicine from Salerno to the Black Death*, ed. L. García-Ballester, R. French, J. Arrizabalaga, and A. Cunningham (Cambridge: Cambridge University Press, 1994), 242–48.

about through other causes, such as rottenness imprisoned in the inner parts of the earth that are released, or already in fact have been released, whenever there are earthquakes. But all of these things which have done and are doing harm, by putrefying the air and water, could have come about through the configurations [of the planets], the aforesaid universal and distant cause.

Concerning Prognostications and Signs.   Changes of the seasons are a great source of plagues. For the Ancients, and especially Hippocrates, are agreed that if any of the four seasons was disrupted so that the seasons did not observe their regularity, pestilence and deadly diseases would come to pass in that year. Therefore we speak from experience when we say that for some time now the seasons have not been regular. For the past winter was less cold than it ought to have been, with much rain, and the spring was windy and, at the tail end, rainy. But the summer was late, less hot than it usually is and extremely wet, very unpredictable from day to day and hour to hour, and the skies often cloudy but then clearing up, so that it seemed as if it was about to rain but it never did. Also, the autumn was very rainy and cloudy. Hence for us, this whole year, or most of that time, has been and still is hot and wet, and for that reason the air is pestilential. For air that is hot and wet does not occur during the seasons of the year except in times of pestilence. . . .

Nevertheless, in the judgment of astrologers who base themselves on Ptolemy,[5] these [plagues] are further reckoned to be likely and possible because there have been seen very many vapor trails and flare-ups, such as a comet and shooting stars. Also, the color of the heavens has customarily appeared yellowish and the sky turned red because of the frequently burnt vapors. In addition, there has been much lightning and frequent flashes, thunder and wind so violent and strong that it has stirred up much of the earth's dust, bringing it from southerly parts. These, especially the powerful earthquakes, quickly make things worse for everyone, leaving behind a legacy of yet more decay, and a multitude of fish, beasts, and other carcasses on the seashore, and also in many places trees covered with dust. And indeed, some confess to have seen a multitude of frogs and snakes, which come forth out of decomposition. All these things seem to come from a great rottenness of the air and land. Moreover, all of the above has been noted before by wise men

---

[5]Claudius Ptolemy (second century CE) was a mathematician and an astronomer in Alexandria.

of worthy memory who made their investigations on the basis of sure experience. . . .

On the other hand, a no small part of the cause of sicknesses is the condition of the patient's body, in that no cause is apt to take effect unless the patient shows a predilection toward it. And it must be particularly emphasized that, although everyone at one time or another incurs the danger of this corrupt air through their necessity to breathe, nevertheless not everyone is made sick by the corruption of the air, but many who are predisposed to it will become [sick]. Truly, those who become sick will not escape, except the very few. Moreover, the bodies that are more susceptible to receive the stamp of this plague are those bodies that are hot and wet, in which decay is more likely. Also [at risk] are: bodies that are full and obstructed with evil humors, in which waste matter is not consumed or expelled as is necessary; that live by a bad regimen, indulging in too much exercise, sex, and bathing; those who are weak and thin and very fearful. Also infants, women, and the young, and those whose bodies are fat and have a ruddy complexion or are choleric are to be on their guard more than others. But those who have bodies that are dry and free of impurities, who govern [their bodies] well and in accordance with a suitable regimen, are more resistant to the pestilence. What is more, we should not neglect to mention that an epidemic always proceeds from the divine will, in which case there is no other counsel except that one should humbly turn to God, even though this does not mean forsaking doctors. For the Most High created medicine here on earth, so that, while God alone heals the sick, He allows medicine as a symbol of his humanity. Blessed be the glorious and high God, who never denies His aid but makes plain to those who fear Him a clear diagnosis for being cured.

8

ALFONSO DE CÓRDOBA

Letter and Regimen concerning the Pestilence

ca. 1348

Little is known about Córdoba. Although he obviously came from Spain, an inscription at the end of his treatise, Epistola et Regimen de Pestilentia *(*Letter and Regimen concerning the Pestilence*), states that it was written at Montpellier in France. No date is given, although it is believed to be either 1348 or 1349. The University of Montpellier was one of the leading medical schools in Europe at the time, and it is clear that Córdoba was connected to it from the way he describes himself at the beginning of his work. Córdoba probably composed his treatise in response to the pronouncement on the plague by the University of Paris in 1348. Rather than positing an astrological or natural cause, like the Paris masters, Córdoba focuses on an artificial or a human one.*

I, Alfonso of Córdoba, master of the liberal and medical arts, have examined with much study the cause and nature of the pestilences which have arisen and begun in the present year of our Lord 1348. The first pestilence was a natural one and its cause was an eclipse of the moon occurring immediately before in the sign of Leo [i.e., July 23–August 22], accompanied by a powerful conjunction of the unlucky planets. The second was caused by a very strong earthquake which many can recall, and that pestilence was naturally located in regions of Italy and in parts overseas, in the corner of the triangle opposite the house of Europe [i.e., an indefinite region to the east]. But that plague ought to have ceased, and so it has ceased, which it did quickly within the space of a year, and otherwise the strength and vigor of the constellation [of the planets] was not in accordance with how it afterwards spread. And yet today the pestilence is spread throughout all the regions of Christendom.

And there is another cause besides the natural one, and for this reason and out of compassion for the [Christian] faithful who chiefly suffer

Karl Sudhoff, "Pestschriften aus den ersten 150 Jahren nach der Epidemie des 'schwarzen Todes' 1348," *Archiv für Geschichte der Medizin* 3 (1909–1910): 224–25.

from it, I have written down this letter and regimen, along with its medicines, so that pious and good people may not be subjected to so many dangers and may know how to prevent the great dangers and evils that especially threaten Christians in this pestilence. Before all else, one must be on one's guard against all food and drink which can be infected and poisoned, especially against non-flowing water, because this can most easily be infected. Experience teaches us that this pestilence does not proceed from some constellation [of the planets] nor as a consequence of any natural infection of the elements, but it proceeds out of a deep-seated malice through the most subtle artifice that can be invented by a profoundly wicked mind.[1] This is why the wise counsel of doctors does not profit or help those in the grip of this most cruel and pernicious disease. Wherefore the best remedy is this: to flee the plague, because the plague does not follow the fugitive, or to take precautions, inasmuch as possible, against infection of all of life's necessities. . . . [Córdoba proceeds to give some recipes for theriacs and electuaries.] The use of such an electuary may preserve one from the venom and poison.

And the use of pestilential pills is of great value, and may preserve one from infected air, because air can be infected by artifice, as when a certain formula is prepared in a glass amphora [flask]. And when that formula is well fermented, he who wishes to do that evil [i.e., poison others] waits until there comes a strong and steady wind from some part of the world. Then he must go against the wind and place his amphora next to some stones opposite the city or town that he wishes to infect. And after giving this area a wide berth, walking away against the wind so that the vapor does not infect him, he should forcefully throw the amphora against the stones, and once the amphora is broken, the vapor spreads and disperses in the air and anyone who comes into contact with that vapor will die as if from pestilential air, and quickly. [Córdoba then gives some more recipes for pestilential pills and recommends fumigating the air with coal fires perfumed by one of the pills.]

---

[1]Jacme d'Agramont also mentions this cause: "Another cause from which plague and pestilence may come is from wicked men, children of the devil, who with venoms and diverse poisons corrupt the foodstuffs with evil skill and malevolent industry."

9

GENTILE DA FOLIGNO

Short Casebook

1348

A physician's son from Foligno, near Perugia in Umbria, Gentile da Foligno was perhaps the most famous and respected doctor in Italy at the time of the Black Death. He studied medicine at the universities of Bologna and Padua. He was a lecturer on medicine at the University of Perugia from 1325 to 1337 and subsequently at Padua until 1345, when he seems to have returned to Perugia. Known for his reliance on practical experience rather than abstract theory when diagnosing or treating diseases, Foligno conducted several public dissections and autopsies, including one at Padua in 1341. He was a prolific writer on a variety of medical topics. His work included commentaries on the entire Canon *of Avicenna, and he wrote a long* Consilium contra Pestilentiam *(Casebook against the Pestilence), which he probably completed before the plague arrived in Italy; three shorter* Consilia *are also attributed to him. Although Foligno's authorship of these short* Consilia *is not universally accepted by scholars, they closely reflect his teaching. The following selection is from the third and last short* Consilium, *addressed to the college of physicians of Perugia and written just before his death, when he had acquired more knowledge about the disease. When plague struck, Foligno bravely resolved to perform his duties. He died of plague on June 18, 1348, apparently having contracted the disease "from too constant attendance on the sick," according to his devoted student, Francesco da Foligno, who attended him at his deathbed and edited this, his last* Consilium.*

Concerning the cause of this pestilence, the view of the masters [of medicine] varies. Certain masters, namely astrologers, say that a solar eclipse that happened many years ago ought to be the cause. Others say that [it is] a great conjunction of Saturn and Jupiter, which occurred in the year of our Lord 1345 in the sign of Aquarius, so that you have an

Karl Sudhoff, "Pestschriften aus den ersten 150 Jahren nach der Epidemie des 'schwarzen Todes' 1348," *Archiv für Geschichte der Medizin* 5 (1911): 83–86.

equal distribution of its effects [here on earth]. Others say that [the pestilence] came to pass from the corruption of the water caused by Saturn in [the sign of] Pisces.

Furthermore, there is this, that the immediate and particular cause is a certain poisonous matter, which is around the heart and lungs and is generated there, whose stamp is not from an excess of any of its qualities, but is due to the nature of the poison [itself]. Thus, wherever poisonous vapors accumulate, a great outbreak of this pestilence arises from the breathing in and imbibing [of these vapors], so that it spreads not only from man to man but also from city to city. . . .[1]

It seems that in times past, there were several wondrous and astounding causes that preceded the pestilence, which now seems to come from southern and eastern parts to Italy, beginning in the west of the country. For the famous pestilence of the city of Crannon,[2] or that which Thucydides or Galen or Avenzoar wrote about, do not seem comparable in their evil to [this] pestilence that has chiefly invaded [Italy].[3] . . .

Therefore, Gentile da Foligno, together with the venerable college of the masters of [the University of] Perugia, prescribed with divine help the following for the preservation and defense against this pestilence:

First, that men should appropriately consume fine food and drink in measured quantities and of suitable quality, and they ought to understand fine food and drink, to which men in general are accustomed. But fish is to be avoided, for on no account should men consume it. Moreover, concerning lettuce, it is advised that if it has been left out in the cold, men should by no means consume it, but that when its color comes back, it is safe to eat. Furthermore, from among various foods, we recommend the eating of good meat, including fowl, chicken, and starlings. But of beef, [we recommend] gelded cows and lactating goats and calves, as well as young pork. Also, we recommend bread carefully prepared and select wines, so that men may live in good cheer as they give vent to their fear.

---

[1] This paragraph is lifted almost word-for-word from Foligno's long *Consilium*; although written well before the Black Death epidemic, it evidently was considered relevant enough for inclusion even after Foligno had personally encountered the plague.

[2] The location of this city is unknown and the reference to plague here is rather mysterious. Avenzoar, or Ibn Zuhr (1090–1162), who was a rival of Avicenna's, also mentions the plague of Crannon.

[3] This represents a significant change from Foligno's position in his first, long *Consilium*: "This said plague seems to grow ever more frightening, although in its malice it is still not so great as that of the city of Crannon which Avenzoar relates in his *Liber Theizir*, or which Thucydides or Galen wrote about."

Second, that one should make use of purgatives and phlebotomies,[4] and larch fungus with its healing properties is always recommended as a purgative, in accordance with what doctors have been prescribing, etc.

Third, that men should take at least two or three times a week until the end of May [1348] the best theriac[5] or antidote. And, if the patient is a man, this should be given to him if he is between the ages of fourteen and thirty-one; it can be given to women in the same doses or more if they are between the ages of fourteen and thirty and a half. Moreover, for babies who are in their first year, who should not take these doses, it will suffice to rub their bodily parts, namely the chest, stomach, and nose, with the theriac. Furthermore, the dose should be taken in the morning with pure wine, or with wine diluted with water, but without drinking the usual refreshments. But the theriac ought to have been already aged for one year, and because not all men can obtain a theriac, it is recommended that poor men consume prasium or hyssop and scabiosa or elecampane, in whatever manner is pleasing to the patient: whether by boiling or liquefying them in wine, or eating them finely chopped, or eating them raw, or drinking wine made from them, or eating them with a little vinegar or wine or with wine only or with water, or drinking their juice. And one can eat only one of the aforementioned things and continue with it, or [eat] one of them in one way and another in a [different] way. Moreover, a dose in any quantity—whether taken once or twice or three times—ought to be sufficient, and these can be useful not only to the poor but also to the rich. But, as for the effectiveness of a theriac, if it is thus given after the aforesaid month [of May], we cannot be the judge.

Fourth, it is recommended that fires be lit in homes and in places where people are living, and that men rest quietly. Also, fires of any kind of fragrant plant should be set up, and the house and city should be cleansed of foul matter [i.e., excrement], and to counteract the foulness, fruits and spices—which are described below—should be at one's disposal.

Lastly, we will respond to questions posed by the common people, and first among these is whether garlic is effective in this pestilence. And it is recommended that ordinary and rustic men, to whom a theriac is not available, may use this, but that others should not. For its intended use

---

[4]"Phlebotomy" is the medical term for bleeding, a practice meant to restore the balance of bodily humors.

[5]A compound of elements used since ancient times and often composed of dozens of ingredients, the most important of which was snakeskin, thought to neutralize the deadly poison inside a sick person. Foligno was a strong advocate of theriac as a cure of plague because he considered the cause of the disease to be poisonous rather than humoral in nature.

is that it be of some effect against disease, but instead during the plague the heart breaks it down into something else, which happens when it is tainted with water.

A second question is whether a compound made of Armenian bole,[6] aloe, myrrh, and saffron be effective in this pestilence, which indeed doctors north of the Alps have prescribed. Our response is that this compound, if prudently made up by doctors in accordance with the conditions of each illness, which may be observed in the patient's members, and even though true [Armenian] bole may not be seen or found in our country, nonetheless if it were to be found and even if it were not genuine, all the same we could accept its use to counteract a certain blocking of the paths of the spirit [i.e., the arteries], which we have found in those men short of breath in the lungs, and because we have found that a tightness of the chest causes harm throughout the body's trunk. But if it should be discovered that the chest is disposed to be tight at certain times, then there is no cause for concern and its use is not recommended.

A third enquiry is whether bitter herbs, vinegar, and verjuice are of any use, and we advise that the vinegar be mixed with wine, provided that the wine is good and the odor is tolerable. But since both will generate heat, it would be safer to use pure vinegar. Moreover, the college recommends that, by the grace of the Lord who is our cure in this, some good men who confer with doctors make regulations for their city, in accordance with [the doctors'] information, so that they safeguard their citizens' well being. All these things, together with many other concerns that we have examined, are elementary to the authors of medical textbooks. But doctors' diagnoses, which are treated in these writings above, may be added to or taken away in accordance with what is found to suit the circumstances of each city and locality and individual person. We pray God that He may improve men's health.

---

[6]Armenian bole is a form of clay high in iron oxide. Galen prescribed it, and it was well known among medical authorities in the Middle East. It was both taken internally and applied externally as a treatment for the bubo swellings.

10

JACME D'AGRAMONT

Regimen of Protection against Epidemics
April 24, 1348

*A physician and professor of medicine at the University of Lérida in
northeastern Spain, Jacme d'Agramont finished composing his work,*
Regiment de preservacio a epidimia o pestilencia e mortaldats *(Regimen of Protection against Epidemics or Pestilence and Mortality), on
April 24, 1348. This makes it the earliest datable plague treatise, and
Agramont himself died from the plague shortly afterward. The* Regimen
*is written in the form of an open letter addressed to the city aldermen
and councillors of Lérida, who commissioned the work. It is obviously
intended for the general public, as it is written in a vernacular tongue,
Catalan, rather than the academic Latin preferred by university scholars.
Nonetheless, Agramont is careful to point out in his introduction that his
work suggests a regimen of prevention only, a very timely one as rumors
of pestilence have come to Lérida from neighboring lands. (Plague was
to hit the region in May 1348.) For treatment of the disease, Agramont
refers the reader to a trained physician and refuses to provide any self-
help tips. Only portions of two of the six sections are included here.*

Rectification of Air, Putrid and Corrupt in Its Substance. If air is pestilential because of putrefaction and corruption of its substance, one must
consider whether its corruption or putrefaction was sent for our deserts
in chastisement for our sins, or whether it came through the infection
of the earth, or of the water, or of allied things, or whether it came from
higher or superior causes such as the influence of conjunctions or appositions of planets. Because if the corruption and putrefaction of the air
has come because of our sins, the remedies of the medical art are of
little value, for only He who binds can unbind. . . .

Jacme d'Agramont, "Regiment de preservacio a epidimia o pestilencia e mortaldats,"
trans. M. L. Duran-Reynals and C.- E. A. Winslow, *Bulletin of the History of Medicine*
23 (1949): 75, 78–85. American Association for the History of Medicine, Johns Hopkins
University. Reproduced with permission of Johns Hopkins University Press, Journals
Publishing Division, via Copyright Clearance Center.

But if the putrefaction of the air came from the earth or from the water, in such case one must choose for one's habitat high places and mountains.[1] But if the putrefaction came through the influence of some conjunction or appositions of the planets, in such case one must choose low places and underground rooms to live in, and also in such cases one must keep windows and embrasures tightly shut.

And one should make fires in the room of good firewood, such as rosemary and myrtle, or of cypress, which one finds in great abundance, or of juniper or Arabic *desticados* [word is unidentified] or of lavender, vulgarly called *espigol*. . . .

[Agramont then gives a special concoction for fumigations by "great lords."] Also one can prepare for the great lords fumigations of a most precious confection which is called *Gallia muscata* [literally, "French musk"], or of another one called "black confection."

But the common folk may use the following regimen. They can make fire in their huts and in their chambers of rosemary and juniper, and make fumigations of incense and myrrh or of other things cheaply to be had such as "cimiama" [cumin] or "herb of thur" [frankincense]. And I will say that the fire alone can effectively rectify air putrid in its substance. I advise that such a regimen be continued as one of the most important and necessary. And again it must be said that it is most beneficial to sprinkle the floor of the room with rose water and vinegar.

Regimen of Exercise. In such times one must avoid violent exercise because such exercise causes much air which is foul and poisoned to be drawn to the heart. The heart is corrupted and also the blood and its spirits, by air that has the effects spoken of in the fourth article [above].

On Foods and Remedies Which Preserve the Body against Pestilential Maladies. The regimen of foods and medicines which are to preserve the body from pestilential maladies must be the following: Man should eat and drink as little as possible. Especially, drinking must be temperate and it is advisable that he control his thirst. Also one should use in all foods much vinegar, sorrel, juice of oranges and of lemons and other acid things which are most beneficial. Clear fresh wine is better

---

[1]Agramont's hometown of Lérida violated this principle; he describes it as "a town which suffers from many maladies . . . although it is on a height and exposed to winds . . . and open to the rising sun," all of which should have cleansed it of the pestilential air. He resolves this dilemma by claiming that diseases in Lérida are "due not to bad air, but to an excessive regimen of fruits and viands, because of their abundance," an ironic viewpoint given his dietary prescriptions.

than sweet wine, because wine that contains sweetness putrefies more easily and has great tendency to turn into bile. Also one must avoid in such times birds that feed near stagnant waters, such as water hens, and geese, and ducks and other animals that have naturally humid flesh, such as suckling pigs and lambs. Also, in such times slimy fishes such as lampreys and eels and rapacious fishes, such as dolphin, shark, tunny-fish, and similar fishes should be forbidden. Especially to be avoided, aside from the above-mentioned fishes, are any others when they are rotten and smelling badly. And if perchance one is obliged to partake of them, one should choose whatever is best in the region, such as salmon, sturgeon, mullets, flounder, and haddock and similar fishes, and they should be preserved in vinegar or salt. Fish fried or grilled over the coals is best in such times.

Of fruits in such times, those are better that are rather acid, such as red berries, acid pomegranates, and *taperes en sols* [capers].

Having pointed out what foods are beneficial, and which are objectionable in such times, we must now mention the medicines which preserve our body from pestilential maladies. One should take three times a week in the morning one drachm or three dinars [the weight of three coins] of fine theriac. It is said to be very beneficial, especially if the body is purged in the manner which we will mention in the following chapter. . . . [Agramont proceeds to give some recipes, including one by Avicenna.]

The Regimen of Sleep.   After feeding naturally follows sleeping. I say that for sleeping there should be selected a room according to the principles discussed in the regimen of air.

Regimen of Our Bodies as Regards Purgation and Bleeding.   Since few are those that in eating and drinking do not go to excess, for this reason I advise that the body be purged with a light purge, i.e. not too strong to be dangerous. . . . [Agramont here gives several recipes for purgative syrups.]

However, since many factors will influence the work of the physician, I advise that in this regimen a good and approved physician be consulted. Because a purge cannot be good at all times nor for everybody, just as one shoe can fit but few.

The desired evacuation having taken place, one can shortly after bleed the median vein or some other in order to withdraw blood, 3 or 4 ounces, more or less according to the condition of the person or according to major or minor necessity. And if one asks me in which quarter of the moon it is best to let blood, I say in the third quarter. And also I say that it is better to do it in the middle of this third quarter, provided that the moon in such times is not seen in a sign unfavorable for bloodletting, such as Gemini, Leo, Virgo, Capricorn, and some others.

And in this regimen it is also important that man abstain from carnal intercourse with woman. To go to excess in these matters is at all times of great danger to our body. But, especially in such times, it does signally and notably great harm and damage.

And also I say that in such times habitual bathing is also very dangerous, because the bath opens the pores of the body and through these pores corrupt air enters and has a powerful influence upon our body and on our humors.

Influences on the Soul: Anger, Joy, Fear, Sadness, Anxiety. I declare that in such times gaiety and joyousness are most profitable, unless joyousness is combined with a bad regimen either of food or of dissipation or other things.

But among other influences that must be avoided in such times are especially those of fear and imagination. For from imagination alone, can come any malady. So one will find that some people get into a consumptive state solely by imagination. This influence is of such great force that it will change the form and figure of the infant in the mother's womb.

And to prove the great efficacy and the great power of imagination over our body and our lives, one can quote in proof first the Holy Scripture, where we read in Genesis, chapter 30, that the sheep and goats that Jacob kept, by imagination and by looking at the boughs which were of divers colors put before them by Jacob when they conceived, gave birth to lambs and kids of divers colors and speckled white and black. Another proof of this proposition can be made by the following experiment: When somebody stands on a level board on the flat floor, he can go from one end to the other with nothing to hold on to, so as not to fall off, but when this same board is placed in a high and perilous position, no one would dare to try to pass over the said board. Evidently the difference is due wholly to the imagination. In the first case there is no fear, and in the other there is. Thus, it is evidently very dangerous and perilous in times of pestilence to imagine death and to have fear. No one, therefore, should give up hope or despair, because such fear only does great damage and no good whatsoever.

For this reason also it is to be recommended that in such times no chimes and bells should toll in case of death, because the sick are subject to evil imaginings when they hear the death bells. . . .

And since in such times maladies and deaths can come from various causes, since it happens that some die from worms and others from abscesses which invade the heart, and others from other causes, it is advisable that in such times, of those that die suddenly, some should be autopsied and examined diligently by the physicians, so that thousands, and more than thousands could benefit by preventive measures against those things which produce the maladies and deaths discussed.

4

Societal and Economic Impact

Undoubtedly, the most searing social experience during the Black Death was the heart-wrenching choice nearly every family must have faced at some point in the epidemic: whether to stay and risk their lives tending their sick loved ones or to flee and save themselves, abandoning those left behind to their fate. Some such complaint is made by no fewer than twenty-one authors writing during the Black Death, including the Florentine humanist Giovanni Boccaccio (Document 12). This dilemma resonated with contemporaries and was not simply a formulaic trope repeated from earlier sources.[1] The temptation to abandon a plague-stricken house or community also meshed well with medieval doctors' advice to "flee quickly and far and return late."[2] Fear of abandonment during plague had far-reaching social implications, such as inspiring a "cult of remembrance," in which patrons sought more individualistic portrayals of themselves for posterity, and more elaborate funeral arrangements and intercessions for their souls in the afterlife.[3] Remarkably, many of the same social and economic responses to the Black Death can be traced in the Muslim Middle East as in Christian Europe (Document 13).[4]

Economically, the Black Death is believed to have delivered the "greatest demand-side shock" (i.e., drastically fewer consumers of food and other goods) and the "greatest supply-side shock" (i.e., fewer laborers available to work) ever recorded in history.[5] This had numerous implications for late medieval economy and society, but historians have identified three main impacts: an increase in real wages for most laborers, such that they now enjoyed a "Golden Age"; the decline and end of serfdom, leading to a more capitalistic system; and greater accessibility to the land market for medieval peasants, with the result that a new social class emerged by the end of the Middle Ages, the yeoman farmer (i.e., someone who farmed 40–100 acres of land).[6] What we focus on here is the labor legislation passed in several countries in Europe in the immediate aftermath of the Black Death—including England, Italy, France, and Spain—in an attempt to fix wages and working conditions to what they had been before the plague epidemic (Documents 14 and 15).[7] In England, we also have court records, such as the assize roll for Wiltshire (Document 16), that can give us some idea of the effectiveness of the labor statute and how vigorously it was enforced and resisted.[8]

NOTES

[1] Paul the Deacon, writing in the eighth century, said of the plague in Italy of 565, that "sons fled, leaving the corpses of their parents unburied," while "parents, forgetful of their duty, abandoned their children in raging fever." Some claim that this inspired Boccaccio's famous account of how "brothers abandoned brothers," and so on, although others argue that chroniclers of the Black Death supply too many original, unique details for them to be merely copying from their ancestors. See Paul the Deacon, *History of the Lombards*, II: 4, trans. William Dudley Foulke (Philadelphia: University of Pennsylvania Press, 1974); Vittore Branca, *Boccaccio Medievale e Nuovi Studi sul Decameron* (Florence: Sansoni, 1956), 381–94; Shona Kelly Wray, "Boccaccio and the Doctors: Medicine and Compassion in the Face of Plague," *Journal of Medieval History* 30 (2004): 303–4; Thomas G. Bergin, *Boccaccio* (New York: Viking Press, 1981), 290; Gabrielle Zanella, "Italia, Francia, e Germania: Una Storiografia a Confronto," in *La Peste Nera: Dati di una Realtà ed Elementi di una Interpretazione* (Spoleto: Centro italiano di studi sull'alto medioevo, 1994), 66–67.

[2] Gentile da Foligno, *Consilium contra pestilentiam* (Colle di Valdelsa, ca. 1479), 5; Karl Sudhoff, "Pestschriften aus den ersten 150 Jahren nach der Epidemie des 'schwarzen Todes' von 1348," *Archiv für Geschichte der Medizin* (hereafter referred to as *AGM*) 4 (1911): 420; *AGM* 8 (1915): 237; *AGM* 14 (1922–1923): 85, 140; *AGM* 16 (1924–1925): 35, 61, 84; *AGM* 17 (1925): 24; R. Simonini, "Il Codice di Mariano di Ser Jacopo sopra 'Rimedi Abili nel Tempo di Pestilenza,'" *Bollettino dell'Istituto Storio Italiano dell'Arte Sanitaria* 9 (1929): 164.

[3] Samuel K. Cohn Jr., *The Cult of Remembrance and the Black Death: Six Renaissance Cities in Central Italy* (Baltimore, Md.: Johns Hopkins University Press, 1997); Samuel K. Cohn Jr., "The Place of the Dead in Flanders and Tuscany: Towards a Comparative History of the Black Death," and Clive Burgess, "'Longing to Be Prayed For': Death and Commemoration in an English Parish in the Later Middle Ages," in *The Place of the Dead: Death and Remembrance in Late Medieval and Early Modern Europe*, ed. Bruce Gordon and Peter Marshall (Cambridge: Cambridge University Press, 2000), 17–65; Eamon Duffy, *The Stripping of the Altars: Traditional Religion in England, 1400–1580* (New Haven, Conn.: Yale University Press, 1992), 301–37.

[4] For an interesting case study comparing the economic impact of the medieval Black Death in Egypt and England, see Stuart J. Borsch, *The Black Death in Egypt and England: A Comparative Study* (Austin: University of Texas Press, 2005).

[5] Bruce M. S. Campbell, "Grain Yields on English Demesnes after the Black Death," and Mark Bailey, "Introduction: England in the Age of the Black Death," in *Town and Countryside in the Age of the Black Death: Essays in Honour of John Hatcher*, ed. Mark Bailey and Stephen Rigby (Turnhout, Belgium: Brepols, 2012), xxxv, 121; Mark Bailey, *The Decline of Serfdom in Late Medieval England: From Bondage to Freedom* (Woodbridge, Suffolk: Boydell Press, 2014), 65.

[6] For some of the main works on these topics, see John Hatcher, "Unreal Wages: Long-Run Living Standards and the 'Golden Age' of the Fifteenth Century," in *Commercial Activity, Markets and Entrepreneurs in the Middle Ages: Essays in Honour of Richard Britnell*, ed. Ben Dodds and Christian D. Liddy (Woodbridge, Suffolk: Boydell Press, 2011), 1–24; Christopher Dyer, "A Golden Age Rediscovered: Labourers' Wages in the Fifteenth Century," in *Money, Prices and Wages: Essays in Honour of Professor Nicholas Mayhew*, ed. Martin Allen and D'Maris Coffman (Basingstoke, Hampshire: Palgrave Macmillan, 2015), 180–95; Bailey, *Decline of Serfdom*; P. D. A. Harvey, ed., *The Peasant Land Market in Medieval*

England (Oxford: Clarendon Press, 1984); Bruce M. S. Campbell, "Population Pressure, Inheritance and the Land Market in a Fourteenth-Century Peasant Community," in *Land, Kinship and Life-Cycle*, ed. Richard M. Smith (Cambridge: Cambridge University Press, 1984), 87–134; Bruce M. S. Campbell, "The Land," in *A Social History of England, 1200– 1500*, ed. Rosemary Horrox and W. Mark Ormrod (Cambridge: Cambridge University Press, 2006), 179–237.

[7]For a European-wide perspective on medieval labor legislation, see Samuel K. Cohn Jr., "After the Black Death: Labour Legislation and Attitudes towards Labour in Late-Medieval Western Europe," *Economic History Review* 60 (2007): 457–85.

[8]For works that focus on the English labor laws, see Bertha Haven Putnam, *The Enforcement of the Statutes of Labourers during the First Decade after the Black Death, 1349–1359* (New York: Columbia University Press, 1908); L. R. Poos, "The Social Context of Statute of Labourers Enforcement," *Law and History Review* 1 (1983): 27–52; Simon A. C. Penn and Christopher Dyer, "Wages and Earnings in Late Medieval England: Evidence from the Enforcement of the Labour Laws," *Economic History Review*, 2nd ser., 43 (1990): 356–76; Chris Given-Wilson, "Service, Serfdom and English Labour Legislation, 1350– 1500," in *Concepts and Patterns of Service in the Later Middle Ages*, ed. Anne Curry and Elizabeth Matthew (Woodbridge, Suffolk: Boydell Press, 2000), 21–37.

11

FRANCESCO PETRARCH

Letters on Familiar Matters

May 1349

One of the giants of early Renaissance Florence, Francesco Petrarch, born in Arezzo in 1304, helped define the emerging spirit of humanism, an intellectual movement that looked back to classical antiquity as the pinnacle of civilization and viewed human endeavors as a fit subject for study. Along with Dante, Villani, and his friend, Boccaccio, Petrarch helped create the first vernacular literature in Italian, although he also wrote extensively in Latin. Yet Petrarch was also firmly rooted in the events of his times, including the Black Death. The following selection is from a letter he wrote from Parma in May 1349 to his friend in Avignon, Louis Sanctus, whom he nicknamed "Socrates." Petrarch laments the effect that plague is having on human friendship. The letter is part of a collection, Epistolae de Rebus Familiaribus *(Letters on Familiar Matters), that he dedicated to Sanctus. Petrarch died in 1374.*

Francesco Petrarch, *Epistolae de Rebus Familiaribus et Variae*, ed. Giuseppe Fracassetti, 3 vols. (Florence: Typis Felicis le Monnier, 1859–1863), 1:438–40, 442–44.

If you wish to bemoan the fates of all mortal men, one breast and one tongue will not suffice for you. You have taken on an enormous, miserable, and irksome subject, useless, inexplicable. Tears must be sought from another source: Indeed, they are always springing up out of some recent and unending cause of sorrow, and the two eyes, already worn out, exhausted and dried up, can pour out only a little melancholy moisture. What therefore can you do to forget, except spread the poison, proffered as medicine, to your friends, not being content with your own misery and sickness, in which you keep knowing and wishing that you would fall? . . .

In the year 1348, one that I deplore, we were deprived not only of our friends but of peoples throughout all the world. If anyone escaped, the following year mowed down others, and whatever had been passed over by the storm, is then pursued by a deadly scythe. When will posterity believe this to have been a time in which nearly the whole world—not just this or that part of the earth—is bereft of inhabitants, without there having occurred a conflagration in the heavens or on land, without wars or other visible disasters? When at any time has such a thing been seen or spoken of? Has what happened in these years ever been read about: empty houses, derelict cities, ruined estates, fields strewn with cadavers, a horrible and vast solitude encompassing the whole world? Consult historians, they are silent; ask physicians, they are stupefied; seek the answer from philosophers, they shrug their shoulders, furrow their brows, and with fingers pressed against their lips, bid you be silent. Will posterity believe these things, when we who have seen it can scarcely believe it, thinking it a dream except that we are awake and see these things with our open eyes, and when we know that what we bemoan is absolutely true, as in a city fully lit by the torches of its funerals we head for home, finding our longed-for security in its emptiness? O happy people of the next generation, who will not know these miseries and most probably will reckon our testimony as a fable!

I do not deny that we deserve these misfortunes and even worse; but our forebears deserved them too, and may posterity not deserve them in turn. Therefore why is it, most Just of judges, why is it that the seething rage of Your vengeance has fallen so particularly hard upon our times? Why is it that in times when guilt was not lacking, the lessons of punishment were withheld? While all have sinned alike, we alone bear the lash. We alone, I say; for I hear it affirmed that compared to the number we receive at present, the lashes inflicted upon all men after that most famous ark [of Noah] had borne the remnants of humanity upon the formless sea would have been a delight, a joke, and a respite. Even when it behooves us to wage countless wars against these evils, in the course of which many kinds of remedies are tried, in the end it is not permitted to men to at least die with dignity. For it is a rare solace of death to die well. No remedy is exactly right, and there is no solace. And to the accumulated disaster is added not knowing the causes and origin of the evil. For neither ignorance nor even the plague itself is more hateful than the nonsense and tall tales of certain men, who profess to know everything but in fact know nothing. Nonetheless their mouths, although accustomed to lying, are in the end silent, and although at first impudence had opened them out of habit, at last they are closed by stupidity.

But I return to my inquiry: Whether for those making a long journey it happens that one part of the way is tiring, another easy. For so it is with us that Your forbearance, God, has slackened little by little toward human crimes, and under the heavy burden of Your yoke, the Omnipotent now must set down His provisions, and You, the best traveler, no longer able to support us, throw us onto Your back and in Your anger avert Your eyes of mercy from us. What if we are making atonement not just for our crimes, but also for those of our fathers, whether these be worse I do not know, but certainly they were more pitiable. Or could it be perhaps that certain great truths are to be held suspect, that God does not care for mortal men? But let us drive these foolish thoughts from our minds. If God did not care for us, there would be nothing left to sustain us. For who will provide these necessities for us, if they are not attributed to God, but to nature; what feeling will be left to us, why give ourselves over to the quest for truth? Since Seneca[1] calls most ungrateful all those who neglect their duties to God, under a different name, are they not denying His due of heavenly majesty by impiously mocking Him? Surely You do care for us and our affairs, God. But there is some reason, hidden and unknown to us, why down through all the ages we, who are the most dignified of Your creatures, seem to be the ones most severely punished. Not that Your justice is less because it is concealed, for the depth of Your judgments is inscrutable and inaccessible to human senses. Therefore either we are truly the worst of all beings, which I would like to deny but dare not, or God is reserving us for some future good the more He is exercising and purging us from these present evils, or there is something there that we are altogether unable to conceive. In any case, whatever the reasons may be and however many are hidden from us, the results are most evident. . . .

---

[1]Lucius Annaeus Seneca, 4 BCE–65 CE, tutor and adviser to Emperor Nero, was an important writer and leading exponent of the Stoic school of philosophy.

Where are our sweet friends now? Where are the beloved faces? Where are the agreeable words, where the soothing and pleasant conversation? What lightning bolt devoured them? What earthquake overturned them? What storm submerged them? What abyss swallowed them? Once we were all together, now we are quite alone. We should make new friends, but where or with whom, when the human race is nearly extinct, and it is predicted that the end of the world is soon at hand? We are—why pretend?—truly alone. . . . You see that our great band of friends is reduced in number. And behold, even as we speak we too are drifting apart, and we vanish like shadows. And in the same moment that one hears that the other is gone, he is soon following in his footsteps. . . .

Never does it seem to me to be a sadder occasion than when one inquires with trepidation after a friend. How goes it? How is our friend doing? But as soon as he has heard you say "farewell," he is filled with dread and very quickly his face is wet with tears. And indeed he—I cannot say this without shedding many tears, and I would shed many now when I say this, except that with all the evil events that have happened these eyes have become exhausted and I would rather save all the rest of my tears, if there are any left, for when they are needed—I say that he is suddenly seized by this pestilential disease, which is now ravaging the world, toward evening, after a dinner with friends and that at sundown he goes to bed, after having digested so much from our conversation in the remembrance of our friendship and our exploits together. He passes that night among his last sorrows in a greatly terrified frame of mind. But in the morning he succumbs to a quick death, and as if this misfortune were not enough, within three days, his sons and all his family follow him.

12

GIOVANNI BOCCACCIO

Introduction to The Decameron
1349–1351

A leading figure of the early Italian Renaissance, Giovanni Boccaccio helped create the first vernacular literature in Italian. He was born in or near Florence, and his father intended him to have a banking career, but eventually Boccaccio devoted himself to writing literature. Although he spent the 1330s in Naples at the court of Robert of Anjou, some scholars believed that Boccaccio came back to Florence in 1341 in time to witness the ravages of the Black Death, which he describes in the introduction to his most famous work, The Decameron, *composed between 1349 and 1351. In this selection, Boccaccio makes a number of striking observations about the way his fellow Florentines responded to the disease: how even close family members changed the way they related to one another; how human responses fell into one of three characteristic behaviors — isolation, denial, and moderation; and how funerals changed as the mortality began to rise. Boccaccio died at Certaldo in 1375.*

Some people were of the opinion that a sober and abstemious mode of living considerably reduced the risk of infection. They therefore formed themselves into groups and lived in isolation from everyone else. Having withdrawn to a comfortable abode where there were no sick persons, they locked themselves in and settled down to a peaceable existence, consuming modest quantities of delicate foods and precious wines and avoiding all excesses. They refrained from speaking to outsiders, refused to receive news of the dead or the sick, and entertained themselves with music and whatever other amusements they were able to devise.

Others took the opposite view, and maintained that an infallible way of warding off this appalling evil was to drink heavily, enjoy life to the full, go round singing and merrymaking, gratify all of one's cravings

---

The Decameron, by Boccaccio, translated by G. H. McWilliam (Penguin Classics 1972, Second edition 1995), 52–57. Copyright © G. H. McWilliam, 1972, 1995. Reproduced by permission of Penguin Books Ltd.

whenever the opportunity offered, and shrug the whole thing off as one enormous joke. Moreover, they practiced what they preached to the best of their ability, for they would visit one tavern after another, drinking all day and night to immoderate excess; or alternatively (and this was their more frequent custom), they would do their drinking in various private houses, but only in the ones where the conversation was restricted to subjects that were pleasant and entertaining. Such places were easy to find, for people behaved as though their days were numbered, and treated their belongings and their own persons with equal abandon. Hence most houses had become common property, and any passing stranger could make himself at home as naturally as though he were the rightful owner. But for all their riotous manner of living, these people always took good care to avoid any contact with the sick.

In the face of so much affliction and misery, all respect for the laws of God and man had virtually broken down and been extinguished in our city [of Florence]. For like everybody else, those ministers and executors of the laws who were not either dead or ill were left with so few subordinates that they were unable to discharge any of their duties. Hence everyone was free to behave as he pleased.

There were many other people who steered a middle course between the two already mentioned, neither restricting their diet to the same degree as the first group, nor indulging so freely as the second in drinking and other forms of wantonness, but simply doing no more than satisfy their appetite. Instead of incarcerating themselves, these people moved about freely, holding in their hands a posy of flowers or fragrant herbs, or one of a wide range of spices, which they applied at frequent intervals to their nostrils, thinking it an excellent idea to fortify the brain with smells of that particular sort; for the stench of dead bodies, sickness, and medicines seemed to fill and pollute the whole of the atmosphere.

Some people, pursuing what was possibly the safer alternative, callously maintained that there was no better or more efficacious remedy against a plague than to run away from it. Swayed by this argument, and sparing no thought for anyone but themselves, large numbers of men and women abandoned their city, their homes, their relatives, their estates and their belongings, and headed for the countryside, either in Florentine territory or, better still, abroad. It was as though they imagined that the wrath of God would not unleash this plague against men for their iniquities irrespective of where they happened to be, but would only be aroused against those who found themselves within the city walls; or possibly they assumed that the whole of the population would be exterminated and that the city's last hour had come.

Of the people who held these various opinions, not all of them died. Nor, however, did they all survive. On the contrary, many of each different persuasion fell ill here, there, and everywhere, and having themselves, when they were fit and well, set an example to those who were as yet unaffected, they languished away with virtually no one to nurse them. It was not merely a question of one citizen avoiding another, and of people almost invariably neglecting their neighbors and rarely or never visiting their relatives, addressing them only from a distance; this scourge had implanted so great a terror in the hearts of men and women that brothers abandoned brothers, uncles their nephews, sisters their brothers, and in many cases wives deserted their husbands. But even worse, and almost incredible, was the fact that fathers and mothers refused to nurse and assist their own children, as though they did not belong to them.

Hence the countless numbers of people who fell ill, both male and female, were entirely dependent upon either the charity of friends (who were few and far between) or the greed of servants, who remained in short supply despite the attraction of high wages out of all proportion to the services they performed. Furthermore, these latter were men and women of coarse intellect and the majority were unused to such duties, and they did little more than hand things to the invalid when asked to do so and watch over him when he was dying. And in performing this kind of service, they frequently lost their lives as well as their earnings.

As a result of this wholesale desertion of the sick by neighbors, relatives, and friends, and in view of the scarcity of servants, there grew up a practice almost never previously heard of, whereby when a woman fell ill, no matter how gracious or beautiful or gently bred she might be, she raised no objection to being attended by a male servant, whether he was young or not. Nor did she have any scruples about showing him every part of her body as freely as she would have displayed it to a woman, provided that the nature of her infirmity required her to do so; and this explains why those women who recovered were possibly less chaste in the period that followed.

Moreover a great many people died who would perhaps have survived had they received some assistance. And hence, what with the lack of appropriate means for tending the sick, and the virulence of the plague, the number of deaths reported in the city whether by day or night was so enormous that it astonished all who heard tell of it, to say nothing of the people who actually witnessed the carnage. And it was perhaps inevitable that among the citizens who survived there arose certain customs that were quite contrary to established tradition.

It had once been customary, as it is again nowadays, for the women relatives and neighbors of a dead man to assemble in his house in order to mourn in the company of the women who had been closest to him; moreover his kinsfolk would forgather in front of his house along with his neighbors and various other citizens, and there would be a contingent of priests, whose numbers varied according to the quality of the deceased; his body would be taken thence to the church in which he had wanted to be buried, being borne on the shoulders of his peers amidst the funeral pomp of candles and dirges. But as the ferocity of the plague began to mount, this practice all but disappeared entirely and was replaced by different customs. For not only did people die without having many women about them, but a great number departed this life without anyone at all to witness their going. Few indeed were those to whom the lamentations and bitter tears of their relatives were accorded; on the contrary, more often than not bereavement was the signal for laughter and witticisms and general jollification—the art of which the women, having for the most part suppressed their feminine concern for the salvation of the souls of the dead, had learned to perfection. Moreover it was rare for the bodies of the dead to be accompanied by more than ten or twelve neighbors to the church, nor were they borne on the shoulders of worthy and honest citizens, but by a kind of gravedigging fraternity, newly come into being and drawn from the lower orders of society. These people assumed the title of sexton, and demanded a fat fee for their services, which consisted in taking up the coffin and hauling it swiftly away, not to the church specified by the dead man in his will, but usually to the nearest at hand. They would be preceded by a group of four or six clerics, who between them carried one or two candles at most, and sometimes none at all. Nor did the priests go to the trouble of pronouncing solemn and lengthy funeral rites, but, with the aid of these so-called sextons, they hastily lowered the body into the nearest empty grave they could find.

As for the common people and a large proportion of the bourgeoisie, they presented a much more pathetic spectacle, for the majority of them were constrained, either by their poverty or the hope of survival, to remain in their houses. Being confined to their own parts of the city, they fell ill daily in their thousands, and since they had no one to assist them or attend to their needs, they inevitably perished almost without exception. Many dropped dead in the open streets, both by day and by night, whilst a great many others, though dying in their own houses, drew their neighbors' attention to the fact more by the smell of their rotting corpses than by any other means. And what with these, and the others who were dying all over the city, bodies were here, there, and everywhere.

Whenever people died, their neighbors nearly always followed a single, set routine, prompted as much by their fear of being contaminated by the decaying corpse as by any charitable feelings they may have entertained toward the deceased. Either on their own, or with the assistance of bearers whenever these were to be had, they extracted the bodies of the dead from their houses and left them lying outside their front doors, where anyone going about the streets, especially in the early morning, could have observed countless numbers of them. Funeral biers would then be sent for, upon which the dead were taken away, though there were some who, for lack of biers, were carried off on plain boards. It was by no means rare for more than one of these biers to be seen with two or three bodies upon it at a time; on the contrary, many were seen to contain a husband and wife, two or three brothers and sisters, a father and son, or some other pair of close relatives. And times without number it happened that two priests would be on their way to bury someone, holding a cross before them, only to find that bearers carrying three or four additional biers would fall in behind them; so that whereas the priests had thought they had only one burial to attend to, they in fact had six or seven, and sometimes more. Even in these circumstances, however, there were no tears or candles or mourners to honor the dead; in fact, no more respect was accorded to dead people than would nowadays be shown toward dead goats. For it was quite apparent that the one thing which, in normal times, no wise man had ever learned to accept with patient resignation (even though it struck so seldom and unobtrusively), had now been brought home to the feeble-minded as well, but the scale of the calamity caused them to regard it with indifference.

Such was the multitude of corpses (of which further consignments were arriving every day and almost by the hour at each of the churches), that there was not sufficient consecrated ground for them to be buried in, especially if each was to have its own plot in accordance with long-established custom. So when all the graves were full, huge trenches were excavated in the churchyards, into which new arrivals were placed in their hundreds, stowed tier upon tier like ships' cargo, each layer of corpses being covered over with a thin layer of soil till the trench was filled to the top. . . .[1]

[1] Another Florentine chronicler, Marchionne di Coppo Stefani, compared the layering of dirt and bodies in mass graves to "how one layers lasagna with cheese."

I must mention that, whilst an ill wind was blowing through Florence itself, the surrounding region was no less badly affected. In the fortified towns, conditions were similar to those in the city itself on a minor scale; but in the scattered hamlets and the countryside proper, the poor unfortunate peasants and their families had no physicians or servants whatever to assist them, and collapsed by the wayside, in their fields, and in their cottages at all hours of the day and night, dying more like animals than human beings. Like the townspeople, they too grew apathetic in their ways, disregarded their affairs, and neglected their possessions. Moreover they all behaved as though each day was to be their last, and far from making provision for the future by tilling their lands, tending their flocks, and adding to their previous labors, they tried in every way they could think of to squander the assets already in their possession. Thus it came about that oxen, asses, sheep, goats, pigs, chickens, and even dogs (for all their deep fidelity to man) were driven away and allowed to roam freely through the fields, where the crops lay abandoned and had not even been reaped, let alone gathered in. And after a whole day's feasting, many of these animals, as though possessing the power of reason, would return glutted in the evening to their own quarters, without any shepherd to guide them.

13

AHMAD IBN ʿALĪ AL-MAQRĪZĪ

A History of the Ayyubids and Mamluks

Fifteenth Century

Ahmad Ibn ʿAlī al-Maqrīzī was born in Cairo, Egypt, in 1364. Following in the footsteps of his father, he pursued a career as an Islamic scholar and administrator until about 1418, when he decided to devote himself to being a full-time historian, perhaps inspired by the example of his friend, Ibn Khaldūn. The following selection concerns the social and economic impact of the Black Death in the Mamluk empire of Egypt and Syria,

Gaston Wiet, "La Grande Peste Noire en Syrie et en Égypte," *Études d'orientalisme dédiées à la mémoire de Lévi-Provençal*, 2 vols. (Paris: G.-P. Maisonneuve et Larose, 1962), 1:375–80.

beginning in January 1349; it is taken from one of al-Maqrīzī's many historical works, kitab al-Sulūk li-maʿrifat duwal al-mulūk *(A History of the Ayyubids and Mamluks). Although al-Maqrīzī was writing more than half a century after the first plague outbreak of 1348, his histories are thought to preserve earlier sources now lost. Al-Maqrīzī died in February 1442.*

In January 1349, there appeared new symptoms that consisted of spitting up of blood. The disease caused one to experience an internal fever, followed by an uncontrollable desire to vomit; then one spat up blood and died. The inhabitants of a house were stricken one after the other, and in one night or two, the dwelling became deserted. Each individual lived with this fixed idea that he was going to die in this way. He prepared for himself a good death by distributing alms; he arranged for scenes of reconciliation and his acts of devotion multiplied. . . .

By January 21, Cairo had become an abandoned desert, and one did not see anyone walking along the streets. A man could go from the Port Zuwayla to Bāb al-Nasr[1] without encountering a living soul. The dead were very numerous, and all the world could think of nothing else. Debris piled up in the streets. People went around with worried faces. Everywhere one heard lamentations, and one could not pass by any house without being overwhelmed by the howling. Cadavers formed a heap on the public highway, funeral processions were so many that they could not file past without bumping into each other, and the dead were transported in some confusion. . . .

One began to have to search for readers of the Koran for funeral ceremonies, and a number of individuals quit their usual occupations in order to recite prayers at the head of funeral processions. In the same way, some people devoted themselves to smearing crypts with plaster; others presented themselves as volunteers to wash the dead or carry them. These latter folk earned substantial salaries. For example, a reader of the Koran took ten *dirhams*.[2] Also, hardly had he reached the oratory when he slipped away very quickly in order to go officiate at a new [funeral]. Porters demanded 6 *dirhams* at the time they were engaged, and then it was necessary to match it [at the grave]. The gravedigger demanded fifty *dirhams* per grave. Most of the rest of these people died without having taken any profit from their gains. . . . Also families

---

[1]This was apparently the busiest boulevard in medieval Cairo.
[2]A *dirham* is a silver coin used in the Muslim world.

kept their dead on the bare ground, due to the impossibility of having them interred. The inhabitants of a house died by the tens and, since there wasn't a litter ready to hand, one had to carry them away in stages. Moreover, some people appropriated for themselves without scruple the immovable and movable goods and cash of their former owners after their demise. But very few lived long enough to profit thereby, and those who remained alive would have been able to do without. . . .

Family festivities and weddings had no more place [in life]. No one issued an invitation to a feast during the whole time of the epidemic, and one did not hear any concert. The *vizier*[3] lifted a third of what he was owed from the woman responsible [for collecting] the tax on singers. The call to prayer was canceled in various places, and in the exact same way, those places [where prayer] was most frequent subsisted on a *muezzin*[4] alone. . . .

The men of the [military] troop and the cultivators took a world of trouble to finish their sowing [of fields]. The plague emerged at the end of the season when the fields were becoming green. How many times did one see a laborer, at Gaza, at Ramleh, and along other points of the Syrian littoral,[5] guide his plow being pulled by oxen suddenly fall down dead, still holding in his hands his plow, while the oxen stood at their place without a conductor.

It was the same in Egypt: When the harvest time came, there remained only a very small number of *fellahs*.[6] The soldiers and their valets left for the harvest and attempted to hire workers, promising them half of the crop, but they could not find anyone to help them reap it. They loaded the grain on their horses, did the mowing themselves, but, being powerless to carry out the greatest portion of the work, they abandoned this enterprise.

The endowments[7] passed rapidly from hand to hand as a consequence of the multiplicity of deaths in the army. Such a concession passed from one to the other until the seventh or eighth holder, to fall finally [into the hands] of artisans, such as tailors, shoemakers, or public criers, and

---

[3]The chief minister of the caliph, or leader of the Muslim community.
[4]An official of the mosque who called the faithful to prayer from the minaret.
[5]The coastal plain of southern Palestine, where the most fertile land was located.
[6]Arabic word for ploughman or tiller, which also denoted the peasantry of Egypt and is the origin of the modern term *fellahin*.
[7]Mamluk commanders and elite soldiers, like their Ayyubid predecessors, were paid out of the revenues of land grants, known as *iqtas* (similar to the fiefs in Europe). With the dearth of labor caused by the Black Death, it became far more difficult to extract income from these estates.

these mounted the horse, donned the [military] headdress, and dressed in military tunics.

Actually, no one collected the whole revenue of his endowment, and a number of holders harvested absolutely nothing. During the flooding of the Nile[8] and the time of the sprouting of vegetation, one could procure a laborer only with difficulty: On half the lands only did the harvest reach maturity. Moreover, there was no one to buy the green clover [as feed] and no one sent their horses to graze over the field. This was the ruin of royal properties in the suburbs of Cairo, like Matarieh, Hums, Siryaqus, and Bahtit. In the canton [administrative district] of Nay and Tanan, 1,500 *feddans*[9] of clover were abandoned where it stood: No one came to buy it, either to pasture their beasts on the place or to gather it into barns and use it as fodder.

The province of Upper Egypt was deserted, in spite of the vast abundance of cultivable terrain. It used to be that, after the land surface was cultivated in the territory of Asyūt,[10] 6,000 individuals were subject to payment of the property tax; now, in the year of the epidemic [1348–1349], one could not count on more than 106 contributors. Nevertheless, during this period, the price of wheat did not rise past fifteen *dirhams* per *ardeb*.[11]

Most of the trades disappeared, for a number of artisans devoted themselves to handling the dead, while the others, no less numerous, occupied themselves in selling off to bidders [the dead's] movable goods and clothing, so well that the price of linen and similar objects fell by a fifth of their real value, at the very least, and still further until one found customers. . . .

Thus the trades disappeared: One could no longer find either a water carrier, or a laundress, or a domestic. The monthly salary of a groom rose from thirty *dirhams* to eighty. A proclamation made in Cairo invited the artisans to take up their old trades, and some of the recalcitrants reformed themselves. Because of the shortage of men and camels, a goatskin of water reached the price of eight *dirhams*, and in order to grind an *ardeb* of wheat, one paid fifteen *dirhams*.

---

[8]This usually took place between September and November of every year.
[9]A *feddan* is equivalent to 1.038 acres.
[10]Located along the Nile in Upper Egypt, about midway between Cairo and Aswan.
[11]An *ardeb* is equivalent to 5.62 bushels.

14

CITY COUNCIL OF SIENA

Ordinance
May 1349

Italian city-states were among the first to enact labor legislation in the wake of the Black Death, some as early as 1348. They typically took a two-pronged approach: on the one hand, attempting to restrict laborers' mobility and curb their demands for higher wages; on the other, trying to attract immigrant labor with the promise of attractive conditions. Siena's labor law is included here; the city-states of Venice, Orvieto, and Pisa, as well as Ragusa (modern-day Dubrovnik), across the Adriatic, enacted similar legislation. It is unclear how successful these laws were: Two other labor measures enacted by Siena, dated September 5, 1348, and October 7, 1350, were not renewed. The following ordinance would have been deliberated and voted on by the commune's city council, which was composed of 300 permanent and 150 rotating members. The ordinance is dated May 1349.

Item, because laborers of the land and those who have been accustomed to work the land or orchards on the farms of the citizens and *districtuales* [inhabitants] of Siena extort and receive great sums and salaries for the daily labor that they do every day, they have totally destroyed and abandoned the farms and estates of the aforesaid citizens and *districtuales*, which is not without great danger to the aforesaid holders of the farms. The aforesaid wise men [of the city council] provide and ordain that everyone, of whatever condition he may be, who labors and is accustomed to labor with his own hands be bound and ought to pay six gold *florins*[1] every year to the commune of Siena on behalf of the lord, unless the said laborer or cultivator works or cultivates with his own hands and

---

[1]The *florin*, or *fiorino d'oro*, was a gold coin issued by the city of Florence beginning in 1252. It was equivalent to one *libra*, or Italian pound, or three to four English shillings.

William M. Bowsky, "The Impact of the Black Death upon Sienese Government and Society," *Speculum* 39 (1964): 26, 145*n*.

labor eight *staios*[2] or works eight *staios* of vineyards or orchards in good faith without fraud according to the customs of a good laborer, which at the very least he is bound to render to the said lord. And that everyone who works for hire or wages with oxen or cows or other kinds of plough-teams be bound and ought to pay twelve gold *florins* every year to the commune of Siena on behalf of and in the name of the lord, always with the exception and proviso that the aforesaid laborers with their beasts work, cultivate, and sow twenty *staios* of land, which at the very least they are bound to render to the said lord. And that . . . the *bargello* [exactor] of the commune of Siena be bound and ought to diligently investigate the aforesaid laborers at least every two months, and those whom he finds to have acted against the present provision of laborers . . . should be fined by the said *bargello* in [the amount of] ten Sienese *lira*.[3] And neverthe-less he [the *bargello*] is bound to pay the said lord. It is declared that laborers should be understood as comprising those who are fifteen years of age and above, up to the age of seventy. And the aforesaid wise men [of the city council] have decreed and ordained that if, after the approval of the present ordinances, any persons from anywhere else than the city and *contado* [district] of Siena wish to come to work at the rate of half or more of the said quantity of land, as is stated above [i.e., four *staios* by hand, ten *staios* with beasts], are not bound to contribute anything [i.e., taxes or services] in that community in which they work or live, and they are to hold and ought to hold this said immunity for five years' time after the approval of the present ordinances.

---

[2]A *staio* was equivalent to about one-third of an acre.
[3]One *lira* was equivalent to 0.32 *florin*.

15

THE CÓRTES OF CASTILE

Ordinance

1351

*In Spain, the córtes of Castile, a form of government like the English par-
liament, was convened under the auspices of the crown and comprised
prelates, noblemen, country squires, and town merchants or councillors
throughout the realm. Scholars dispute the exact role of representative
assemblies in Spain's medieval political history: At certain times, for
example, during the 1350s and 1360s in the kingdom of Aragon and
during the 1380s and 1390s in Castile, the córtes demonstrated impressive consultative, legislative, and financial powers on a par with those
of England. But at other times, the córtes met infrequently and was
fragmented among regional assemblies along the model of France. The
following selection describes labor legislation enacted in response to the
Black Death by the córtes convoked by King Pedro I "the Cruel" of Castile
(ca. 1334–1369) at Valladolid in 1351. The córtes of Aragon passed similar decrees in 1350 (subsequently revoked in 1352). The ordinances of
Castile were tailored to each part of the kingdom, suggesting that plague's
impact varied considerably by region. Only the first four ordinances, common to all regions of the kingdom, are included here.*

There have been rumors and complaints made to me [Pedro I of Cas-
tile] that some persons of my land and of my realms suffer very great
losses because they cannot work their estates to produce bread and
wine and other things that maintain men. And this has come about, on
the one hand because many men and women wander about idle and do
not want to work, and on the other because those who do work demand
such great prices and salaries and wages, that those who have estates
cannot comply, and for this reason, these estates have become deserted
and lack laborers. And also there have been rumors and complaints
made to me that those laborers who work and perform other trades

Córtes de los antiguos reinos de León y de Castilla, 5 vols. (Madrid: Real Academia de la
Historia, 1861–1903), 2:75–77.

[that produce things] for the maintenance of men which they cannot go without, sell things from their trades at their will and for much greater prices than they are worth; and from this situation ensue and arise very great damages to all those who have to buy those things that they need. And I, seeing that this has been to my disservice and great damage and loss in all of my land and seeking and desiring the common welfare of those who live in my realms, deem it good to command that an ordinance be made in each of the regions of my realms concerning these matters, in the manner given here.

First, I deem it good and I command that no man nor woman who is fit and able to work wander about idle through my dominions, neither asking [for things] nor begging, but that all work hard and live by the labor of their hands, except those men and women who become so sick and injured or are of such great age that they cannot do anything and boys and girls of twelve years of age [or younger].

Also, I deem it good and I command that all the laboring men and women and persons who can and ought to earn a living, as is said above, continue to perform the same work on the estates and serve for the salaries and wages at the prices contained below, and the same applies to those who are idle.

Also, I deem it good and I command that all the carpenters and builders and plasterers and servants and workmen and workwomen and day laborers and other workers who are accustomed to hire out their labor go to the public square of each place where they live and have been accustomed to be hired at daybreak of every day, [bringing] with them their implements and their food in a manner such that they can go out of the town or place to perform their labor where they were hired at sunrise, and that they work the whole day. And they are to quit their work at such a time that they return to the town or place where they were hired at sunset. And those who work in the town or place where they were hired are to work from the said time of sunrise, and they are to quit working at sunset.

Also, I deem it good and I command that all the laborers continue to work and employ themselves in the professions that they know and are accustomed to, and that they sell the things that they make in their trades and professions for the prices that are contained and given below. And they are to perform the work of their professions well and faithfully.

16

Wiltshire, England, Assize Roll of Labor Offenders

June 11, 1352

The following selection is from an assize court roll, or record of the jury trial that decided cases on a given date, which took place at Devizes, Wiltshire, before three deputy justices of laborers on June 11, 1352, against offenders from the Kingsbridge hundred. (A hundred was a territorial unit of the shire, roughly equivalent in modern terms to a ward in a county.) It provides an example of the way the English government prosecuted offenders of the Statute of Laborers shortly after it was enacted in February 1351. The statute, following upon an ordinance of 1349, decreed that servants and hired laborers must accept the salaries and wages that they had received in 1346, and on that basis it established set wage rates for each category of worker. Moreover, craftsmen and artisans were to charge the same prices they had charged in 1346. Six hundred forty-two people were prosecuted in the county in 1352 for violating the statute. They were drawn from no less than forty-five different occupations, including both agricultural workers and artisans. The government generally prosecuted agricultural workers for wage violations, and artisans for charging excessive prices. Some offenders practiced more than one trade. Undoubtedly, the profession most represented was brewers or tapsters, who made up 24 percent of the offenders and were overwhelmingly female. Only one man, William Spendlove of Eton, was prosecuted for enticing another into his service with promise of higher wages. The following selection comes from the end of the roll, which provides more detail about the cases, including judgments that were handed down (included here in abridged form).

John Laurok came to Chisledon, a vagabond out of service, and pleaded guilty to leaving the service of William de Stratton of Oxfordshire. He is let out on bail and fined six pence.

E. M. Thompson, "Offenders against the Statute of Labourers in Wiltshire, AD 1349," *The Wiltshire Archaeological and Natural History Magazine* 33 (1903–1904): 404–7.

William le Coupere [Cooper] of Elcombe, who at another time before the aforesaid justices swore to exercise his trade in accordance with the Statute [of Labourers of 1351], took an extra six pence for his work from various men contrary to his oath. He pleads not guilty and is acquitted by a jury of twelve men.

John Boltash, carter of the parson of Elingdon [Wroughton], pleads guilty to receiving for his livery [upkeep] two bushels of wheat per quarter of grain for ten weeks [of work], whereas he used to be given one bushel of wheat per quarter for eleven weeks. Walter Clement, oxherd of the same parson, pleads guilty to receiving for his livery this year two bushels of wheat per quarter for ten weeks, whereas he used to be given one bushel of wheat per quarter for eleven weeks. Walter Ryche pleads guilty to receiving from the same parson for his livery two bushels of wheat per quarter for twelve weeks, whereas he used to be given no wheat per quarter for twelve weeks. They are let out on bail to appear at the next session. . . .

Edward le Taillour of Wootton Bassett, servant of the prior and convent of Bradenstoke, made an agreement with them to receive his usual diet and salary from Michaelmas [September 29] 1351 until the Michaelmas following but left their service before the feast of St. Nicholas [December 6, 1351] without leave or reasonable cause contrary to the Statute. His arrest is ordered to the bailiff. . . .

Richard the Cobbler of Clack Mount, who at another time swore to exercise his craft in accordance with the Statute, took an extra forty pence from various men for shoes sold by him contrary to the Statute and his oath. Previously, Richard did not appear before the justices because the bailiff answered that he could not be found. Then, when the bailiff tried to arrest him, Richard took flight upon seeing the bailiff and would not halt. Afterwards, Richard was arrested and brought before the justices and additionally charged with contempt of court. Richard pleads innocent but places himself at the mercy of the court and is fined two marks [twenty-six shillings and eight pence]. . . .

Thomas Tonkere of Calne, a fuller, took an extra twelve pence from various men for his trade contrary to the Statute. He does not appear before the justices because the bailiff answers that he cannot be found. He is to be arrested and brought to the next session and is fined in absentia twelve pence. . . .

Edith Paiers, Alice Dounames, Edith Lange, and Isabel Purs of Clyffe Pypard took an extra six pence last autumn from various men for reaping corn into sheaves. They are let out on bail and fined six pence each.

Walter Cook and his wife Agnes, Thomas Averil and his wife Alice, and John London of Thornhill took an extra six pence from various men for reaping corn last autumn contrary to the Statute. They plead guilty and are let out on bail. Cook is fined twelve shillings, while Averil and London are fined twelve pence each.

Thomas, formerly the servant of Ralph de Chusleden, left Ralph's service without reasonable cause before the end of the term agreed upon between them and refused to serve anymore contrary to the Statute. Thomas does not appear before the justices because the bailiff answers that he cannot be found. He is to be arrested and brought to the next session.

John, a shepherd of Walter Halman of Medbourne, took from Walter for his livery two bushels of wheat per quarter of corn for a half-year [of work] instead of two bushels of barley, worth an extra twenty pence. John pleads guilty and is let out on bail and fined two shillings [twenty-four pence].

5

Religious Mentalities

Religion was central to the medieval European response to the Black Death. For Christians, plague was proof of the righteous judgment of God visited upon a sinful humanity, yet there was still hope that God's vengeance may be appeased by prayers, processions, and other appeals directed to saints with special intercessory power (Document 17). In addition, plague created some logistical problems for the Church, such as finding enough priests to service parishes, particularly the poorer ones decimated by the disease that could now barely provide a living from oblations and tithes (Documents 18 and 19).

For Muslims, plague was believed to be a mercy and a martyrdom for believers that came directly from God.[1] Nonetheless, the denizens of the Islamic Middle East likewise sought to appease God with prayers and processions to try to ward off the Black Death (Document 20). Yet, Muslim religious ideas about plague seemed to preclude secondary or intermediate causes of disease, such as contagion; Christian doctors, by contrast, widely accepted and promulgated the concept of contagion, with no apparent objections from the Church. Muslim doctors who championed contagion, such as Lisān al-Dīn Ibn al-Khatīb (Document 21), had to contend with *fatwas*, or religious teachings, like those issued by the fourteenth-century Grenadan jurist, Abu Sa'id Faraj Ibn Lubb, which hewed to the traditional line that there was no contagion and that one should not flee from a plague-infected region. Lubb's objection to flight was also based on the concept that a Muslim had a social obligation to his fellow Muslim and should stay by his side to attend to him in his illness.[2] Those who believed in contagion, however, were more likely to abandon the sick to die of hunger and thirst, as indeed was complained of by many Christian authors (Chapter 4).

Nonetheless, the prophetic tradition of Islam was not inveterately hostile to contagion, and there was a long tradition of accommodating empirical approaches, particularly those derived from the ancient Greeks and Romans, with the faith. This would indicate that any differences between Christians and Muslims with respect to their views on plague were one of degree, rather than one of outright acceptance or rejection of any given concept. Still, these differences may have become magnified later, in the fifteenth century, when Islam turned more decisively against contagion under the influence of the Egyptian scholar Ibn Hajar al-'Asqalānī.[3] Meanwhile, in Christian Europe, many towns embraced plague-control measures, such as quarantine, even when these conflicted with religious responses, such as public processions.[4]

NOTES

[1]Michael W. Dols, *The Black Death in the Middle East* (Princeton, N.J.: Princeton University Press, 1977), 109; Michael W. Dols, "The Comparative Communal Responses to the Black Death in Muslim and Christian Societies," *Viator* 5 (1974): 275; Lawrence I. Conrad, "Epidemic Disease in Formal and Popular Thought in Early Islamic Society," in *Epidemics and Ideas: Essays on the Historical Perception of Pestilence*, ed. T. Ranger and P. Slack (Cambridge: Cambridge University Press, 1992), 77–99.

[2]Justin K. Stearns, *Infectious Ideas: Contagion in Premodern Islamic and Christian Thought in the Western Mediterranean* (Baltimore, Md.: Johns Hopkins University Press, 2011), 79–85, 115–20.

[3]Ibid., 69–79, 85–89.

[4]Carlo M. Cipolla, *Public Health and the Medical Profession in the Renaissance* (Cambridge: Cambridge University Press, 1976), 11–66; Carlo M. Cipolla, *Faith, Reason, and the Plague in Seventeenth-Century Tuscany*, trans. M. Kittel (Ithaca, N.Y.: Cornell University Press, 1979), 1–14; Ann G. Carmichael, *Plague and the Poor in Renaissance Florence* (Cambridge: Cambridge University Press, 1986), 98–126; Neil Murphy, "Plague Ordinances and the Management of Infectious Diseases in Northern French Towns, c. 1450–c. 1560," in *The Fifteenth Century, XII: Society in an Age of Plague*, ed. Linda Clark and Carole Rawcliffe (Cambridge: Cambridge University Press, 2013), 139–59; Carole Rawcliffe, *Urban Bodies: Communal Health in Late Medieval English Towns and Cities* (Woodbridge, Suffolk: Boydell Press, 2013); Kristy Wilson Bowers, *Plague and Public Health in Early Modern Seville* (Rochester, N.Y.: University of Rochester Press, 2013).

17

MICHELE DA PIAZZA

Chronicle

1347–1361

A Franciscan friar in the convent of Catania in Sicily, Michele da Piazza records perhaps the first arrival of plague on European soil, in October 1347 at Messina. In this selection, Piazza testifies to the powerful appeal

Michele da Piazza, *Cronaca*, ed. Antonino Giuffrida (Palermo: ILA Palma, 1980), 82–87.

of local religious shrines, such as those of the blessed Virgin Agatha of Catania and the blessed Virgin Mary of Santa Maria della Scala, toward which large numbers of people turned for succor, spiritual and otherwise, during the plague epidemic. Piazza reports that supplications to these shrines were accompanied by incidents of the marvelous, although none of them involved healing. At the same time, Piazza also records the rancorous secular rivalries that existed between the Sicilian towns of Messina and Catania, which evidently persisted even at the height of the plague epidemic and from which not even Piazza, a Franciscan friar, could disentangle himself.

Wherefore the Messinese, taking stock of this terrible and monstrous calamity, chose to leave the city rather than stay there to die; and not only did they refuse to enter the city, but even to go near it. They camped out with their families in the open air and in the vineyards outside the city. But some, and they were the majority of the citizens, went to the city of Catania, believing that the Blessed Virgin Agatha of Catania would deliver them from this illness. . . . Indeed, very many Messinese were staying in the city of Catania, where with one voice they implored the lord patriarch through the pious petitions submitted to him, that for the sake of devotion he go personally to Messina, bringing with him with all due honor some of the relics of the Virgin Agatha. "For we believe," they said, "that with the arrival of the relics, the city of Messina will be completely delivered from this sickness." So the patriarch, deeply moved by their prayers, agreed to go personally to Messina with the aforesaid relics. And this was around the end of the month of November in the year of our Lord 1347. The holy Virgin Agatha, seeing through the inward deceit and stratagems of the Messinese—who have always wanted to keep the virgin's relics at Messina and were exploiting the situation for that end—prayed to the Lord to see to it that the whole populace of the city betake themselves to the patriarch, shouting and saying that such a plan in no way pleased them. And wresting the keys away from the churchwarden, they soundly rebuked the patriarch, asserting that he should choose death before agreeing to transfer the relics to Messina. After this scolding, the patriarch could do nothing else but enter the place where the relics were kept in a spirit of great devotion and honor, accompanied by a monastic choir intoning religious chants and holy prayers, and lave [bathe] the holy relics with some pure water; it was this holy water which he arranged to be brought to the city of Messina, when he personally crossed over to there by ship. But oh, what a foolish idea you Messinese had, to think you could steal away the relics of the Blessed Virgin Agatha in this secret manner, under cover of a zealous devotion. Have you forgotten that when the body of the virgin was at Constantinople and desired to go back to her own country, to the city of Catania, she appeared in dreams to Gislebert and Goselin and ordered them to bring her body back to the city of Catania?[1] Don't you know that if she had wanted to make her home in Messina, she by all means would have allowed this to happen? What more is there to say? Afterwards, the patriarch came to the city of Messina, bringing with him the aforesaid holy water, and he cured many and various sick people by sprinkling and touching them with the water. Therefore the citizens of Messina flocked to the patriarch, rushing to see him with great joy and giving many thanks to him and to God. For demons appeared in the city, having changed themselves into the shape of dogs, and they inflicted much harm on the bodies of the Messinese. Struck numb with terror, no one dared leave their homes. Nevertheless, by the general agreement of all and following the wishes of the archbishop of Messina, the citizens resolved to devoutly process around the city while chanting litanies. And as the whole populace of Messina was entering the city, a black dog carrying a drawn sword in its paw appeared among them; growling, it rushed the crowd and broke silver vessels, lamps, and candelabra that were on the altars, and shattered various other kinds of things. At this sight, everyone all at once fell flat on their faces, half-dead with fear. But after a while the men recovered and got up, and they saw the dog leave the church, but no one dared follow it or approach it.

But the Messinese were terrified by this extraordinary vision, so that they all grew fearful to a marvelous degree. Therefore they decided to all walk barefoot in a priest-led procession to the [shrine of the] blessed Virgin [Mary] of Santa Maria della Scala, six miles away from Messina. When they drew near to the Virgin, everyone all at once became transfixed, and on bended knee with tears in their eyes they called with great devotion upon God and the blessed Virgin for aid. And they entered the church saying devout prayers, while the priests chanted the psalm, *misere nostri Deus* (Lord have mercy), and laid their hands upon the sculpted image of the mother of God, set up there since ancient times. They decided to bring this image back to the city of Messina, because they reckoned

---

[1]This is a rather hypocritical passage, considering that Agatha's body often changed hands. Agatha was a third-century Christian martyr from Catania or Palermo, and her relics were removed to Constantinople during the ninth century when Sicily was conquered by the Muslims. In 1126, Gislebert and Goselin stole them and took them back to Catania.

that with it they could rid the city of demonic visions and apparitions, and completely deliver it from this mortality. Accordingly, they chose a suitable priest to honorably carry the image in his arms while riding on his horse. And as they were going back to the city with the aforesaid image, the holy mother of God, when she saw and approached the city, judged it to be loathsome and totally bloodied with sin, so that she turned her back on it and not only refused to enter the city but averted her eyes from it. As a result the earth opened wide, and the horse, upon which the image of the mother of God was being carried, remained fixed and immovable like a rock, unable to go forwards or back. When the people of Messina witnessed this miracle, they gasped with a sharp intake of breath, and weeping copious tears, they prayed to the blessed Virgin to not take new vengeance for their past sins; added to these humble prayers were the sacred entreaties which the holy bride of Christ, the Virgin herself, addressed to the Lord. Whereupon the earth that at first had opened is closed, and the horse moves: but when she came to the city gate, the holy mother of God refused to enter it in any way. Finally, after pious prayers were addressed to her, she entered the great church of the city of Messina, namely the Santa Maria la Nuova. The women of Messina showered the image with silk cloth and precious jewels. But could not the holy mother of God have remained in her church and completely refused to enter the city? Or are we perhaps suggesting that she could be carried away from her station, albeit unwilling? In truth, she could have remained in her original location, because no amount of force could bear her away, she to whom God's power granted all mercy, all might, all goodness. But was this not to terrify the people so that out of fear they might completely purge themselves of their worldly temptations? What more is there to say? The arrival of the image availed nothing; on the contrary, the mortality entrenched itself even further, so that there was nothing else that could be done.

SIMON ISLIP, ARCHBISHOP OF CANTERBURY

Effrenata (Unbridled)

May 28, 1350

From August 1348 to August 1349, England saw the passing of three archbishops of Canterbury: the first victim, John Stratford, probably died of old age in August 1348, but John Offord and Thomas Bradwardine died of plague in May and August 1349, respectively. Simon Islip, who succeeded Bradwardine, endured longer as archbishop, surviving until 1366. The document printed here is from Islip's constitution, Effrenata *(Unbridled), issued on May 28, 1350, to the bishops of the southern province of England. Islip tried to do for the clergy what the ordinance of laborers did for peasant opportunists, that is, to stop parish priests from leaving their churches to work for more lucrative salaries elsewhere, especially in private chapels, or chantries.*

The unbridled greed of the human race would, out of its innate malice, grow to the point that charity would be banished from the bounds of the earth, unless its momentum was checked by the power of justice. Well, the [House of] Commons have brought to us their complaint, and experience, that effective teacher, shows us that surviving priests, who are unmindful of the fact that divine intervention spared them from the recent pestilence—not by reason of their own merits—but so that they can carry out the ministry that was committed to them on behalf of God's people and the public welfare, and who do not blush for shame when their insatiable greed provides a wicked and pernicious example for other workers, even among the laity, now have no regard for the care of souls, which is most worthy of attention from the Church's ministers and which can merit glory to the unwilling man who takes it up, even if he should miserably fail in the rest of his duties. But priests are unwilling to take on the care of souls and to bear the burdens of their cures in mutual charity, but rather they wholly abandon these to devote

Registrum Simonis de Sudbiria Diocesis Londoniensis, AD 1362–1375, ed. R. C. Fowler, 2 vols. (Canterbury and York Society, 34, 38, 1927–1938), 1:190–92.

themselves to celebrating anniversary masses and other private services. So that they can more easily revive old extravagances, they are not content with being paid ordinary salaries but demand for their services excessive wages, and thus they win more profit for themselves than curates do, in exchange only for their status and little work. Unless their unreasonable appetite is reduced to equitable levels, the greater number of anniversary masses and the size of their salaries, moderated by no sense of balance, will mean more and more churches, prebends, and chapels throughout our province, and in our diocese as well as yours, left wholly destitute of the services of priests, and what adds to our sorrow, curates, attracted by similar wages, will be easily distracted toward these same private services, completely abandoning their cures. Wishing therefore to rein in the insatiable desire of these priests, on account of the above perils and other losses which could arise if we did not apply appropriate remedies, we require and exhort you, father, in the bowels of Jesus Christ, that, paying heed to the danger to souls and other causes mentioned above, you suitably provide before all else for the good governance of parish churches, prebends, and chapels whose care of souls is in jeopardy and in accordance with their needs, appointing for them the better and more qualified chaplains that can be found in service to anyone other than a parish. And you are to use whatever censures are sanctioned by the Church in order to act against those who do not comply and against their patrons and those who retain their services despite our ordinance and against all those who have the temerity to violate the ordinance, so that chaplains and anyone else performing any kind of religious service anywhere in your diocese may be content with a moderate salary. And if anyone who defies you seeks on that account to have himself transferred to our diocese or to the diocese of a fellow bishop, we will and order you to make his first and last name known to us through your letters, or to the bishop into whose diocese he has transferred, and inform us of what actions you or your officials have taken against him. For we wish to follow up the actions that you or a fellow bishop has taken against those who come into our diocese, and to execute to the full force of the law the censures that have been inflicted upon them. We require and order that this likewise be done and carried out by all our fellow bishops in their dioceses. And so that it may be clear to you what level of salary has been fixed by us, we have ordained for our diocese [of Canterbury] that chaplains of a parish church, prebend, or chapel with a cure of souls be content to be paid a salary of one mark [just over half a pound] beyond what was formerly accustomed to be paid to a priest with the same cure of souls, but otherwise we wish that the salary of stipendiary priests be limited to the going rate that was in force in times past.

19

HAMO HETHE, BISHOP OF ROCHESTER, AND THOMAS DE LISLE, BISHOP OF ELY

Post-Plague Parish Poverty

July 1, 1349, and September 20, 1349

The following two selections from the registers of Hamo Hethe, bishop of Rochester, and Thomas de Lisle, bishop of Ely, illustrate alternative responses to the death of parishioners from plague, and the attendant falling off of priests' income from their oblations or offerings. Most of a parish priest's income came from the "voluntary" contributions of parishioners, which paid for his services at baptisms, last rites, marriages, confessions, and communions; in addition, parishioners were expected to tithe, or contribute a tenth of their produce, to the church every year. In the second document, the granter of the annual sustenance is John de Oo, who was acting as Thomas de Lisle's vicar-general while the bishop was away on a pilgrimage to Rome. The beneficiaries of the sustenance were two Cambridge priests. The excerpts are dated, respectively, July 1, 1349, and September 20, 1349.

Hamo Hethe, Bishop of Rochester

[July 1, 1349]   Several priests and clerics refuse to accept benefices when these are lawfully offered to them, benefices where the curates have been forced to leave,[1] or even those that are well and truly vacant.

---

[1]The exact term used here is *exilia* or, literally, "exiled." Use of this word suggests that priests have abandoned their parishes out of financial necessity, rather than fear of plague.

Registrum Hamonis Hethe, Diocesis Roffensis, AD 1319–1352, ed. Charles Johnson, 2 vols. (Canterbury and York Society, 48, 1948), 2:886; Cambridge University Library, Ely Diocesan Records; G/I/1, Register Thomas de Lisle, fol. 27v.

Moreover, in some of these benefices the priests are still absent, and have been for a long time, on account of the fact that by now it is well known that their incomes have been diminished by the mortality of the parishioners in these places, so that no one can live or support himself on what is left. We have learned that in many places where this has happened, the parish churches have for a long time remained unserved, and the cures [of souls] there are in danger of being almost abandoned, to the grave peril of souls. We, wishing to apply a remedy for this in so far as we are able right now, concede and grant by the tenor of these presents to all and several rectors and vicars already instituted or about to be instituted in our city and diocese, who have been forced to leave their benefices and whose annual income is ten marks [approximately six and a half pounds] or less, that each of them, while his poverty lasts, can licitly celebrate, or cause to be celebrated, by himself or another, one anniversary mass per year, or any number of masses whose total value equals it, on behalf of his parishioners or patrons from anywhere else outside the diocese, so long as the anniversary masses are celebrated in the parish church in which he was instituted. This is to last until we see fit to decree otherwise.

Thomas de Lisle, Bishop of Ely

[September 20, 1349]   A clear, urgent necessity demands that we provide you with pious aid. We are fully informed by your ample accounts and by the testimony of other trustworthy people that a portion is allotted to you in the aforesaid church from the oblations [offerings] — in so far as these are known — of its parishioners, and that the same parishioners have in the meantime suffered for so long from the pestilence, which is well known to be taking hold in this year, so that the oblations accruing from the said church are by no means sufficient for the necessities of your life, nor can you obtain these elsewhere to allow you to support the burdens incumbent [upon your office]. For this reason you have humbly petitioned us to have an annual sustenance for the necessities of your life for two years. Truly, because it is not seemly for a person of your status in the holy Church of God to beg for life's necessities, such as these consist in your food and clothing, we, by the authority and office of the said father [Bishop Thomas de Lisle], grant that the support be awarded to you, in accordance with what you have requested. Nevertheless, we enjoin through these presents that as soon as you are able to be supported at a suitable level of your necessities through the proceeds and income of your portion, you altogether desist from the

collection of this annual [sustenance], which you are strictly bound to do by virtue of the obedience that you have sworn to the said father.

20

ʿIMĀD AL-DĪN ABŪ 'L-FIDĀ' ISMĀʿĪL B. ʿUMAR IBN KATHĪR

The Beginning and End: On History
ca. 1350–1351

ʿImād al-Dīn Abū 'l-Fidā' Ismāʿīl b. ʿUmar Ibn Kathīr, born in Syria in 1300, was in a good position to observe the religious effects of plague in Damascus. In February 1348, just a few months before the Black Death arrived, he was appointed teacher of the hadith, *or religious traditions relating to Muhammad, at one of the city's religious schools. This excerpt comes from Kathīr's* al-Bidāya wa-ʿl-nihāya fī 'l-tārīkh *(* The Beginning and End: On History*), at the end of which is a chronicle of Damascus. Kathīr died in February 1374.*

At Damascus, a reading of the *Traditions* of Bukhārī[1] took place on June 5 of this year [1348] after the public prayer—with the great magistrates there assisting, in the presence of a very dense crowd—the ceremony continued with a recitation of a section of the Koran, and the people poured out their supplications that the city be spared the plague. Indeed, the population of Damascus had learned that the epidemic extended over the [Syrian] littoral and various points of the province, so that it was predicted and feared that it would become a menace to Damascus, and several inhabitants of the city had already been victims of the disease.

---

[1]Al-Bukhārī, who lived in the ninth century, was a famous collector of Islamic traditions. The work being read from is undoubtedly al-Bukhārī's *Sahih*, a collection of more than 7,000 traditions on a variety of subjects, including the creation, heaven and hell, and the Prophet Muhammad. According to al-Maqrīzī, the reading took place at the Omayyad Mosque and lasted three days and nights.

Gaston Wiet, "La Grande Peste Noire en Syrie et en Égypte," *Études d'Orientalisme dédiées à la mémoire de Lévi-Provençal*, 2 vols. (Paris: G.-P. Maisonneuve et Larose, 1962), 1:381–83.

On the morning of June 7, the crowd reassembled before the *mihrab*[2] of the Companions of the Prophet, and it resumed the recitation of the flood of Noah, of which a reading was made 3,363 times, in accordance with the counsel of a man to whom the Prophet had appeared in song and had suggested this prayer.[3] During this month [of June], the mortality increased among the population of Damascus, until it reached a daily average of more than 100 persons. . . .

On Monday, July 21, a proclamation made in the city invited the population to fast for three days; they were further asked to go on the fourth day, a Friday, to the Mosque of the Foot in order to humbly beseech God to take away this plague. Most of the Damascenes fasted, several passed the night in the mosque indulging in acts of devotion, conforming to the ritual of the month of Ramadan.[4] On the morning of July 25, the inhabitants threw themselves [into these ceremonies] at every opportunity from "every precipitous passage":[5] One saw in this multitude Jews, Christians, Samaritans, old men, old women, young children, poor men, emirs, notables, magistrates, who processed after the morning prayer, not ceasing to chant their prayers until daybreak. That was a memorable ceremony. . . .

On Monday, October 5, after the call to afternoon prayer, a violent storm broke over Damascus and its environs, stirring up a very thick cloud of dust. The atmosphere became yellowish, then black and was totally dark. The population was in a state of anguish for about a quarter of an hour, imploring God, asking His pardon and lamenting all the more that it was afflicted by this cruel mortality. Others imagined that this cataclysm marked the end of their misfortunes, but they did not dwell too much on this. Indeed, the number of cadavers brought to the Omayyad

[2]An arched niche used for prayer, which pointed in the direction of Mecca.

[3]More details of this story are given by al-Maqrīzī, according to whom the holy man came "from the mountains of Asia Minor" and first communicated his vision to the great *qadi*, or judge, of Damascus. His instructions were to "read 3,360 times the flood of Noah and ask God to end this plague that afflicts you." Al-Maqrīzī reports that the Damascenes carried out the holy man's instructions "in a perfect spirit of humility and with an intense repentance of their past sins"; they also allegedly sacrificed a "great number" of sheep and cattle, whose meat was distributed to the poor. After this went on for a week, al-Maqrīzī claims, the plague began to "diminish daily" before disappearing from Damascus entirely. This conflicts with Kathīr's testimony.

[4]One of the five pillars of Islam, fasting during the sacred month of Ramadan is prescribed by the Koran and usually takes place in October and November.

[5]This seems to be a quotation from Koran 22:27: "And proclaim the Pilgrimage among men: They will come to thee on foot and [mounted] on every kind of camel, lean on account of journeys through deep and distant mountain highways." The twenty-second *sura*, or chapter, is on pilgrimage, so this is Kathīr's way of saying that the Damascenes embarked on a plague procession.

Mosque exceeded the figure of 150, without including the dead in the suburbs, and the non-Muslim dead. Now, in the environs of the capital, the dead were innumerable, a thousand in a few days.

21

LISĀN AL-DĪN IBN AL-KHATĪB

A Very Useful Inquiry into the Horrible Sickness
1349–1352

A Muslim scholar and physician, Lisān al-Dīn Ibn al-Khatīb hailed from Loja, a town near Granada, the capital city of an important and tena-cious Moorish kingdom in southern Spain. A friend of Ibn Khatīma, al-Khatīb wrote his own medical account of the plague, titled Muqni^cat as-sā'il ^can al-marad al-hā'il *(A Very Useful Inquiry into the Horrible Sickness). Since he incorporated Ibn Battūta's famous description of the plague epidemic in Southeast Asia, al-Khatīb likely wrote his treatise during his friend's visit to Granada between 1349 and 1352. In this selec-tion, al-Khatīb explains why he rejects the Islamic religious proscription against plague contagion, which was well documented by physicians. His outspokenness against a long-established* hadith, *or religious tradition, backed up by the Shari'a, or Muslim law, was perhaps triggered by the fact that his friend, Khātima, felt compelled to bow to Islamic precept despite empirical observation on the same subject in his own treatise (Docu-ment 6). Al-Khatīb's brave defense of contagion may have contributed to his forced exile from Granada in 1371, when proceedings began for his trial for heresy on the basis of his writings. Before the trial could begin, however, a mob broke into his prison at Fez and lynched him in 1374.*

If it were asked, how do we submit to the theory of contagion, when already the divine law has refuted the notion of contagion, we will answer: The existence of contagion has been proved by experience, deduction,

M. J. Müller, "Ibnulkhatīb's Bericht über die Pest," *Sitzungsberichte der Königl: Bayer-ischen Akademie der Wissenchaften* 2 (1863): 2–12. Translated from the Arabic with assistance from Walid Saleh.

the senses, observation, and by unanimous reports, and these aforementioned categories are the demonstrations of proof. And it is not a secret to whoever has looked into this matter or has come to be aware of it that those who come into contact with [plague] patients mostly die, while those who do not come into contact survive. Moreover, disease occurs in a household or neighborhood because of the mere presence of a contagious dress or utensil; even a [contaminated] earring has been known to kill whoever wears it and his whole household. And when it happens in a city, it starts in one house and then affects the visitors of the house, then the neighbors, the relatives, and other visitors until it spreads throughout the city. And coastal cities are free of the disease until it comes from the sea through a visitor from another city that has the disease, and thus the appearance of the disease in the safe city coincides with the arrival of this man from the contagious city. And the safety of those who have gone into isolation is demonstrated by the example of the ascetic, Ibn Abū Madyan, who lived in the city of Salé [unidentified]. He believed in contagion, and so he hoarded food and bricked up the door on his family (and his family was large!), and the city was obliterated by the plague and not one soul [except Madyan] was left in that whole town. And reports were unanimous that isolated places that have no roads to them and are not frequented by people have escaped unscathed from the plague. And let me tell you of the miraculous survival in our time of the Muslim prisoners who were spared in the prison of the city of Seville, and they were in the thousands. They were not struck by the bubonic plague, yet it almost obliterated the city. And it has been confirmed that nomads and tent dwellers in Africa and other nomadic places have escaped unscathed because their air is not enclosed and it is improbable that it can be corrupted.

And amidst the horrible afflictions that the plague has imposed upon the people, God has afflicted the people with some learned religious scholars who issue *fatwas*[1] [against fleeing the plague], so that the quills with which the scholars wrote these *fatwas* were like swords upon which the Muslims died. . . . Although the intent of the divine law is innocent of harm, when a prophetic statement is contradicted by the senses and observation, it is incumbent upon us to interpret it in a way so that the *hadith* fits reality, even if we claim to subscribe to the literal meaning of the *hadith* and, lest we forget, to the fundamentals of the *Shari'a* [Islamic law] that everybody knows about. And the truth of this matter is that it should be interpreted in accordance with those who affirm the theory of contagion. Moreover, there are in the divine law many indications that

---

[1]A ruling or an opinion based on Islamic law handed down by a qualified legal scholar.

support the theory of contagion, such as the statement of Muhammad: "A disease should not visit a healthy man," or the statement that: "One escapes the fate of God to meet the fate of God." But this is not the place to go on at length concerning this matter, because the discussion about whether the divine law agrees or disagrees with the contagion theory is not the business of the medical art, but is incidental to it. And in conclusion, to ignore the proofs for plague contagion is an indecency and an affront to God and holds cheap the lives of Muslims. And some of the learned holy men have retracted their *fatwas* for fear of helping people to their deaths.

May God keep us from committing error in word and deed!

6

The Plague Psyche

THE FLAGELLANTS

In both popular culture and academic studies, the flagellants—a penitential movement that arose during the Black Death primarily in northern Europe—have the reputation of having been hysterical religious fanatics or radicals, who were hostile to the Church clergy and hierarchy, contributed to attacks against the Jews, and flirted with heresy and apocalyptic tendencies.[1] This is largely a reflection of contemporary views of the flagellants, as detailed in chronicle accounts, such as that by Fritsche Closener of Strasbourg (Document 23). But is this how the flagellants actually saw themselves?

This chapter presents new evidence that may shed light on this problem. It comes in the form of a flagellant scroll dating to 1349 in Middle Dutch, which would have been rolled up and carried from place to place to be read from or consulted as the flagellants performed their distinctive rituals, or ceremonies (Document 22). The discovery and publication of the flagellant scroll opens a new chapter in the history and interpretation of the flagellant movement during the Black Death. For one thing, the scroll shows the flagellants to have been a disciplined group, whose rituals were highly choreographed; thus, any emotional responses to the flagellants, such as recorded by chroniclers, were not spontaneous but carefully solicited by the flagellants themselves. Second, a comparison of the flagellant scroll with chronicles recording the earlier phase of the movement in Germany reveals a high degree of consistency and uniformity in the rituals, which argues against a chronological or temporal evolution of the flagellants toward a more "radical" phase.[2] Third, the scroll makes it clear that the main purpose behind the flagellant movement was its redemptive power to appease God's wrath in order to take away plague. What happened when the Black Death came or remained despite the flagellants' extraordinary penance is, no doubt, bound up with the final suppression of the movement.

22

A Middle Dutch Flagellant Scroll

1349

*In 1994, a medieval document that had been lost since 1917 was redis-
covered and then published in 2003, which represents a milestone in
studies of the flagellants during the Black Death. This is an original
scroll, measuring 3½ inches (91–95 mm) wide and approximately 8 feet
(248.5 cm) long, comprising four strips of parchment of unequal lengths
sewn together. The scroll, which is dated to about 1349 on paleographical
grounds, was designed to be rolled up tightly into a ball that could conveniently be carried in a travel pouch and then taken out to be read during
flagellant ceremonies. Since the language of the scroll is medieval Dutch,
it likely was used by flagellants traveling through the Low Countries,
although much of the scroll seems to have been copied from a German
original. Aside from being a unique document, since only a handful of
such scrolls survive from the Middle Ages, the significance of the scroll
lies in the fact that, for the first time, we have a complete flagellant ritual
(referring to the entirety of the flagellant ceremonies) in its original form.
This allows the flagellants to speak to us directly, in their own voice unfiltered by the usual histories derived from chronicles and other writings
about the flagellants, as represented in Documents 23–24. The flagellant
ritual as depicted on the scroll is divided into three parts: a liturgy; a
"Mary-song"; and a sermon. Only the liturgy is given here, as it seems to
be the most original part of the ritual and the only one during which the
flagellants performed their whipping ceremonies. The liturgy was sung in
the style of a church litany, familiar to all churchgoers of the Middle Ages,
whereby two or three "precentors" would sing one or two verses on their
own, followed by all the flagellants then repeating the verses in unison
before the precentors moved on to the next verses, and so on.*

Who shall do his [Lucifer's] evil will,
He shall pay for it and be forgiven.
Thus his soul will be saved.

Ria Jansen-Sieben and Hans van Dijk, "Un slaet u zeere doer Cristus eere! Het flagellantenritueel op een Middelnederlandse tekstrol," *Ons Geestelijk Erf* 77 (2003): 149–54.

Help, lord God, because it is near to us all.
Come to us, dear lord God,
So that we will fulfill Your command.

Now enters here the penance will,
So that we can flee the hot hell.
Lucifer is an evil companion.
Whom he likes, he nourishes with pitch.
So flee him or you will be his.

Jesus Christ was taken prisoner,
To a cross he was hung.
This cross turned red from blood.
We lament God's martyr and His death.

Sinner, how shall you reward me:
Three nails and a crown of thorns?
On the cross put a spear in me.
Sinner, this I suffer all because of you.
How do you want to suffer than through me?

So we then loudly call:
Accept our services with which here we pay
Shelter us from hell,
So we pray, through Your death.

Because of God we spill our blood.
So that it will precede the sins.
Help us, Mary, queen,
That we will win your Child's praise.

Mary, pure queen,
Through your sweet Child's love,
All our needs are lamented to you.
This comes to us, mother, pure virgin.

The earth trembles, also it tore stones.[1]
Hard hearts, you shall weep.
All in your eyes, Christ's virtues,
All in your heart, Christ grieves.

---

[1]This was perhaps a reference to the Friuli earthquake that occurred on January 25, 1348, and which is discussed by Konrad of Megenberg in Document 29.

Now flail yourself heavily for Christ's honor!
Through God now leave your sins behind.
Through God now let your vainglory go.
So that God will want to protect us.

Now help us, Mary, queen,
That we will win your Child's praise.

Mary stood in great need,[2]
When she saw her sweet Child dead,
A sword that cut all through her heart.
Sinner, let this be your suffering.

Jesus called in a loud voice
On the cross (his death was grim):
"Sinner, I so long after you!"

Jesus was nourished with gall.
This is why we all crosswise fall.[3]

+ + +

Now raise up all your hands,[4]
That God may avert the great death!
Now stretch out all your arms,
That God protect us all!

Jesus, through all your names three
Make us from all sins free!
Jesus, through all your wounds red
Shelter us from the [sudden] death!

[We pray] that He send us His Ghost
And consent to do this shortly.
So help us, Mary, queen,
That we will win your Child's praise!

---

[2]These next four verses were inspired by the *Stabat Mater* hymn from the thirteenth century. According to the chronicler Fritsche Closener (Document 23), this is when the flagellants began to whip themselves, and they continued to do so through at least the next five verses.

[3]This was the signal for all the flagellants to stop their whipping and fall flat on the ground, their arms outspread in the shape of a cross. Three circled crosses were drawn in red at this part of the scroll.

[4]The flagellants at this point apparently got back up again and assumed a kneeling position for the next twelve verses.

Women and men, you have to break off [adulterous relations],[5]
Or God will avenge himself over you.
Sulfur, pitch and also the gall
Pours the devil into you all.

For certain, [adulterers] are the devil's scorn.
Preserve us from this, lord God!
The [marital] law is a pure life,
That God has given us!

I counsel you, women and men all,
Through God now let the vainglory fall!
This the poor soul bids you,
Through God now let the vainglory be spent!
Through God now let the vainglory go!
Thus God will protect us.

Christ called in the kingdom of heaven
His angels all equal:
"Christendom wants to flee me,
This is why I want the world to end
This is for certain, without delusion."

Mary bade her Child so well:
"Sweet Child, let them repent!
Thus I want to pray that they must
Convert themselves. Child, this I pray thee."

You, liar; you, bad caretaker,
Reason is too heavy [a burden] for you.
He who will mourn for his sins,
In new joy he shall trust.

Now confess yourself clean. Leave be delusion,
Thus God will want to renew him then.

Mary stood in great need,
When she saw her sweet Child dead,
A sword that cut all through her heart.
Sinner, let this be your suffering.

---

[5]This marks the start of the flagellants' "Confession," whereby all the flagellants lie down and make a sign befitting their respective sins.

Jesus called in a loud voice
On the cross (His death was grim):
"Sinner, I so long after you!"

Jesus was nourished with gall.
This is why we all crosswise fall.

+ + +

Now raise up all your hands,
That God may avert the great death!
Now stretch out all your arms,
That God protect us all!

Jesus, through all your names three
Make us from all sins free!
Jesus, through all your wounds red
Shelter us from the [sudden] death!

[We pray] that He send us His Ghost
And consent to do this shortly.
So help us, Mary, queen,
That we will win your Child's praise!

Woe to thee, poor usurer,[6]
The scales are too heavy for you.
You set the lot at a pound,[7]
This will sink you in hell's ground.

You, murderer; you, extortionist,
You are by God despised.
You do not want to take care of anyone,
Not of rich, not of poor.
This is why you are lost forever.

Therefore shelter us from this, lord God,
This we pray through Your death.

And if this penance is not found,
The world will altogether sink.
Mary, your hand makes us free.
Sinner, I tell you the happy news.

---

[6]This signaled another Confession sequence, where the flagellants all lay down and made a sign befitting their respective sins.

[7]The "lot" (*lood* in Dutch) was an old unit of measurement that normally was equivalent to 1/30 or 1/32 of a pound.

Saint Peter is a gatekeeper.
Get to him, he will let you in
And bring you to the queen.

Well, lovely angel, Saint Michael,
You are an angel of all souls.
Shelter us from hell,
This is done through your Creator's death.

Help us, Mary, queen,
That we will win your Child's praise!

In short time, God is wrathful,
[Against] him who does not want to celebrate His Sunday,
He must end up in the pains of hell
[And] be bounded like Lucifer.

Therefore, shelter us, lord God,
This we pray thee, through Your death.
Shelter us from hell.

Whoever does not fast on Fridays,
He must rest in hell.

Therefore, shelter us, lord God,
This we pray thee, through Your death.
By God now fast on Friday forevermore,
This we pray thee, you poor soul.

Mary stood in great need,
When she saw her sweet child dead,
A sword that cut all through her heart.
Sinner, let this be your suffering.

Jesus called in a loud voice
On the cross (His death was grim):
"Sinner, I so long after you!"

Jesus was nourished with gall.
This is why we all crosswise fall.

+ + +

Now raise up all your hands,
That God may avert the great death!
Now stretch out all your arms,
That God protect us all!

Jesus, through all your names three
Make us from all sins free!
Jesus, through all your wounds red
Shelter us from the [sudden] death!

[We pray] that He send us His Ghost
And consents to do this shortly.
So help us, Mary, queen,
That we will win your Child's praise!

23

FRITSCHE CLOSENER

Chronicle

1360–1362

The Chronicle *of Fritsche Closener, like that of Giovanni Villani (Document 3), is an early example of municipal history entirely devoted to the author's native or adopted city—in this case, Strasbourg—that was to come into vogue toward the end of the fourteenth century. Closener was born into a noble family from Alsace, and his father is described as a bourgeois of Strasbourg. Ordained as a priest, Closener was appointed prebend of the chapel of St. Catherine in the cathedral of Strasbourg in 1340. He began writing his* Chronicle *in 1360 and, by his own account, completed it on July 8, 1362. Closener's history of the flagellants in Strasbourg is much more detailed than that of his contemporary, Matthias of Neuenburg, who also concerned himself with events related to Strasbourg.*

In 1349, fourteen days after midsummer [July 8], around mass time, about 200 flagellants came to Strasbourg,[1] who carried on in the manner I'm about to describe. First, they had the most precious flags of velvet cloth, rough and smooth, and the finest canopies, of which they had

[1]Matthias of Neuenburg says that seven hundred flagellants came to Strasbourg from Swabia in the middle of June.

Chroniken der deutschen Städte vom 14 bis 16 Jahrhundert. Volume 8: Die Chroniken der oberrheinischen Städte, Strassburg, 2 vols. (Leipzig: S. Hirzel, 1870–1871), 1:105–20.

maybe ten or eight, and torches and many candles, which were carried ahead of them when they went into cities or villages. And all bells were rung in alarm then, and they followed their flags two by two in a row, and they were all wearing overcoats and hoods with red crosses. And two or four sang the beginning of a hymn, and the others joined in. . . . [The hymn begins: "Now the journey has become so grand/Christ Himself rides into Jerusalem."] And when they entered the churches, they knelt down and sang: "Jesus was fortified with gall/That's why we should be on the cross all." With these words they prostrated themselves in the form of a cross, so that it rang out. After they'd been thus for awhile, the lead singer began and sang: "Now we lift up our hands and pray/O God take the great death away!" Then they got up. They did this for three hours. When they had risen for the third time, the people invited the brothers—one invited twenty, another twelve or ten, each one as they could—and they led them to their homes and did them well.

Now this was their rule. Whoever wanted to join the brotherhood had to stay with it for thirty-three and a half days, and for that reason, he had to have so many pennies that he could offer four on every day while he was doing penance: This amounted to eleven shillings and four pence. This was why they did not ask or beg of any one, nor enter any house. When they came to a city or village, they were invited and taken in without their asking. After that, they might enter houses as long as they were in the city. They also were not allowed to speak to any woman.[2] If one broke this rule and spoke to a woman, he knelt in front of their master and confessed. Then the master set the penalty and whipped him with the scourge on his back and spoke: "Rise up from the cleansing pain/ And stay away from sin from now on." They also had a rule that priests may be among them, but none of them should be a master nor belong to their secret council.

When they wanted to do penance, which was at least twice a day, in the morning and at night, they took their scourges and went outside the city limits. While one rang the bells, they gathered and went out in rows of two by two and sang their hymn as described earlier. And when they arrived at the place for whipping, they undressed to their underclothes and barefeet and wrapped little skirts or white cloths about them, which went from the belt to their feet. And when they were ready to begin their penance, they laid down in a wide circle, and whoever had sinned

---

[2]This is contradicted by an anonymous chronicler from the monastery of St. Truiden in the Low Countries, who claims that a breakaway sect of the flagellants "was secretly lodged in the house of a woman across the Rhine." If this is true, it is surprising that Closener does not mention it, especially because it occurred in his vicinity.

laid down anyway, but if there was a villain who had broken his oath, he laid down on one side and raised three fingers and his head, and if there was one who had broken his troth, he laid on his belly. This way, they laid down in many ways, according to the sins which everyone had committed. After they all had lain down, the master began where he saw fit and stepped over one of them and hit his back with the scourge and said: "Rise up from the cleansing pain/And stay away from sin from now on." Thus he walked about them all, and the ones he stepped over followed the master across those who were still down. Thus, when two of them had walked over the third, that one rose and walked with them to the fourth, and the fourth across the fifth one in front of him. They all followed what the master did with the scourge using the same words, until all of them had gotten up and walked over each other. And when they had risen into their circle, some of them, who were considered the best singers, began to sing a hymn. The brothers sang after them, in the same manner as one sings for a dance. All the time the brothers walked in the circle two by two and whipped themselves with the scourges, which had knots at the end into which thorns had been placed, and they whipped themselves across their backs so that many of them were bleeding a lot. . . .

The flagellants' sermon:[3] This is the message of our Lord Jesus Christ, who came down to the altar of the Good Lord St. Peter in Jerusalem, as written on a marble tablet from which a light issued forth, like lightning. God's angel set up this table. The congregation saw this and people fell on their faces and cried "Kyrie eleison," which means "Lord have mercy." The message of our Lord is this:

"You children of men, you have seen and heard what I've forbidden and you didn't heed it, so that you're sinful and unbelieving, and you didn't keep my holy Sunday. And you have not repented and improved, even though you heard in the gospel: 'Heaven and Earth shall perish, but my word stands forever.' I sent you enough grain, oil, and wine,[4] in good measure, and I took it all away in front of your eyes because of

---

[3]Other versions of this sermon occur in the Middle Dutch flagellant scroll and in a letter said to have been delivered by the flagellants of Mechelen to the bishop of Cambrai, as recorded in a contemporary French chronicle. The sermon was not original to the flagellants, but was simply another version of the "heavenly letter," which circulated in various forms since 1200. See Jansen-Sieben and Van Dijk, "Het flagellantenritueel," 169–81; *Corpus Documentorum Inquisitionis Haereticae Pravitatis Neerlandicae*, ed. Paul Frédéricq, 3 vols. (Ghent: J. Vuylsteke, 1889–1906), 3:22–23; Robert E. Lerner, "The Black Death and Western European Eschatological Mentalities," *American Historical Review* 86 (1981): 536–37.

[4]A reference to Joel 1:10. In this case, Israel's abundance was taken away by war.

your wickedness and your sins and pride, because you didn't observe my holy Sunday and my holy Friday, with fasts and celebration. This is why I ordered the Saracens and other heathens that they shed your blood and take many of you prisoners. In a few years, much misery happened: earthquakes, hunger, fever, locusts, rats, mice, vermin, pocks, frost, thunder, lightning, and much disorder. I sent you all this because you haven't observed my holy Sunday. . . .

"I swear to you upon My right hand, that is, by My godly might and by My power: If you don't keep My holy Sunday and My holy Friday, I shall spoil you totally so that no one will ever think of you ever on this earth. Verily, I say: If you reform from your sins, I shall send you My holy divine blessing so that the earth shall bear fruit full of mercy and all the world shall be full of my power. I shall have you partake in My great joy, so that you can sally forth anew and will forget My anger against you and shall fill all your houses with My divine blessing. And when you come before My judgment, I shall share My pity with you, the selected ones in My heavenly empire. Amen. . . ."

Then the people saw the tablet on which was the message light up the domed church just like lightning. At that, the people took fright, so much so that they fell on their face and when they came to, what did they do? They separated and took counsel among themselves as to what they could do to better praise God so that He would overlook His anger. They deliberated and went to the king of Sicily[5] and asked him for his advice as to what they could do to make God amend His anger against them. He told them that they should fall on their knees and pray to Almighty God that He tell them what they should do and how to come to terms with Him so that He would forget His anger against all the poor of Christendom. The people did as they were told and fell on their knees and prayed from the bottom of their hearts. Then the angel said: "You know that God walked on earth for thirty-three and a half years[6] and never had a good day, not to mention the great torture He suffered from you on the cross, for which you never thanked Him and won't thank Him either. If you want to make your peace with God, you should go on a pilgrimage for thirty-three and a half days and should never have a good day nor night and spill your blood. Then He will not want to have His blood lost upon you and He intends to forget His anger against poor

[5]Assuming that this part of the letter is contemporary with the Black Death, this would be Louis the Great of Hungary (r. 1342–1382), who in 1348 led a crusade to Naples and declared himself king of Sicily and Jerusalem.
[6]The age traditionally ascribed to Christ at his crucifixion.

Christendom." . . . [The pilgrimage started by the king of Sicily spread to Poland, Hungary, the German towns, and eventually to the Rhineland and Alsace.]

Thus ended the letter. When it had been read, they returned to the city, two by two, following their flags and candles, and sang the first hymn: "Now is the first pilgrimage." And they rang the big bells for them, and when they came to the main church, they fell down in the shape of a cross and three stood as has been written. When they rose again, they went to their shelters or wherever they wanted to go. . . .

You should know that whenever the flagellants whipped themselves, there were large crowds and the greatest pious weeping that one should ever see. When they read the letter, there rose great lamentation from the people, because they all believed it was true. And when the priests said, how one should recognize that their whipping pilgrimage was the right one, they answered and spoke: "Who wrote the gospels?" Thus they make the people believe the flagellants' word more than those of the priests. And the people spoke to the priests: "What can you say? These are people who know the truth and tell it." And wherever they came, many people of the cities also became flagellants, both laymen and priests, but no learned priest joined them.[7] Many well-meaning men joined this whipping pilgrimage; in their simple-minded way, they could not see the falsehood which resided therein. But also, many a proved scoundrel joined these well-meaning people, who then turned nasty, or nastier than before. Some of them who remained were also well-meaning, but there were not many of them. Some loved the brotherhood very much; after they had done it twice, they started again. For this reason, it happened that when they were on the road, they were idle and didn't work. And wherever they came, as many as they were, people invited them all and gave them everything, and there were many people who liked to invite them, as many of them as they could, they were that highly esteemed.

The burghers in the cities gave them money from the city coffers so that they could buy flags and candles. The [flagellant] brothers also assumed great holiness and said that great things were happening by their will. First, they said, a well-meaning man gave them drink from a barrel of wine, and no matter how many of them drank from it, it was full. They also said that a martyr's image in Offenburg had sweated, and

---

[7]According to Matthias of Neuenburg, one thousand people in Strasbourg joined the flagellants. Nonetheless, he goes on to say that the citizens and burghermeisters, or city councillors, of the city were "divided in opinion about the flagellants, one faction against them, another for them."

that a statue of Our Lady also had been sweating. Thus they said many things, which were all lies. They also said that cattle in Ersthein had been talking. It came about thus: There was someone in Ersthein whose name was Rinder [German word for "cattle"] who was very ill and couldn't speak. It came to pass that the flagellants were there so that the man got better and talked. One said to the other, "Rinder is talking." So the flagellants spoke as if the cattle in the stables had been talking. This shows how simple-minded the country was and the people in it. They also took it upon themselves to exorcize the mad people. . . . They also dragged a dead child about in a meadow around their ring as they whipped themselves and wanted to make it live again, but that didn't happen.

These whipping pilgrimages lasted for more than a quarter of a year, so that every week there was another band of flagellants. Then also women took off and wandered through the land and whipped themselves. Then also young boys and children took up the flagellants' pilgrimage. After that, the people did not want to ring bells for them anymore, and they didn't want to give them any more contributions for candles and flags. One also got tired of them, so that one didn't invite them into homes as one had done before. Thus they became a nuisance and one paid but little attention to them. Then the priests attacked the falsehoods and lies they were spreading around, and they said that the letter was a lie they were preaching. At first, the flagellants had brought the people to their side so much that no one dared speak out against them anymore. Any priest who spoke against them could hardly save himself from the people. But then their pilgrimages didn't go so well, and the priests spoke against them all over again. . . . It was forbidden them to form a brotherhood and whip themselves in public. If one wanted to whip himself, he had to do it secretly in his house. Bishop Berthold of Bucheck also forbade them in his bishopric [of Strasbourg] upon holy orders from the pope, who instructed the bishops that the seemingly spiritual beliefs they held, especially that one layman could confess to another, should be abandoned.

This I have described as it happened, and it was the same in towns all along the Rhine and in Swabia, Franconia, in the West and in many German lands. Thus, the flagellants' pilgrimages ended in half a year, but as they had said, it should have lasted thirty-three and a half years.

24

JEAN DE FAYT

Sermon on the Flagellants
October 5, 1349

*Jean de Fayt, a Benedictine monk and doctor of theology at the Univer-
sity of Paris, was sent by the Paris Theology Faculty to preach a sermon
against the flagellants before Pope Clement VI at Avignon, which he did
on October 5, 1349. Two weeks later, on October 20, Pope Clement issued
his bull suppressing the flagellant movement,* Inter Sollicitudines. *Fayt's
sermon is therefore extremely valuable for the window it provides into the
thinking about, and prejudices against, the flagellants by Church authorities. A native of Flanders, Fayt served as an eyewitness to flagellant ceremonies there, which makes his testimony credible in this respect. But
some of his charges, such as that the flagellants were involved in perse-
cutions of Jews in Germany, can be demonstrated on the basis of other
sources to be suspect and, therefore, seem to be derived from nothing more
than popular hearsay. In true academic fashion, Fayt quotes plentifully
from Scripture and classical authors in support of his position; such quo-
tations are generally omitted from this excerpt.*

Furthermore, most holy father [i.e., Pope Clement VI], . . . a certain
great and arduous business has recently emerged. Indeed, a new sect
of men called the Flagellants has arisen, which adheres to new rules
and ceremonies, that is, singular observances concerning the faith. This
sect or, rather, superstition, already has grown and spread throughout
so many provinces of Christendom that, speaking in the exaggerated
language one frequently encounters in Scripture to convey a great
quantity or multitude, it can truly be said that it has now reached all
the provinces of Christendom.[1] But truly, most holy father, ever since

---

[1]This is manifestly incorrect. There is little evidence, for example, that the flagellants were present in the Mediterranean regions, such as Spain, southern France, and
Italy, even though a flagellant movement did arise in central and northern Italy nearly
a century earlier, in 1260. Flagellants are said to have reached England by the end of

---

Corpus Documentorum Inquisitionis Haereticae Pravitatis Neerlandicae, ed. Paul Frédéricq, 3 vols. (Ghent: J. Vuylsteke, 1889–1906), 3:31–37.

this superstition has recently come as far as the lower parts of France, several bishops and princes, not knowing whose lands [the flagellants] had invaded, are very confused as to what should be done in this business: whether the Flagellants should be allowed to do what they want, or whether they should be resisted by means of ecclesiastical censure as well as by the secular arm. The University of Paris, which, as Peter of Blois testifies in a certain letter,[2] illuminated difficult questions on the most intricate problems, decreed through letters and messengers that the faculty of theology should chiefly advise [on this matter]. But the Paris masters [of theology], reckoning that this business was extremely great and arduous—both because there was a copious multitude adhering to this sect, as well as because there was an unheard of novelty about this sect and its observances, from which Church rites seemed to be threatened with great upheaval—decided by unanimous consent that this business ought to be presented before Your Holiness. Like a high prince, you preside over the entire Church, and, in order that they might act with more decorum, the aforementioned masters humbly beseeched the most illustrious prince, the king of France, that he see fit to communicate with Your Holiness on this business. Indeed, the king, like the zealous Catholic prince that he is of the Christian religion and faith, complied forthwith with their request. Therefore, the king and masters decided to communicate with Your Holiness on this matter through me, although unworthy of so great a commission, since I had come to know about the aforesaid sect [of the flagellants] with my own eyes. They enjoined me to more fully expound on this business to Your Holiness, which, in order that I might do so, I have set this as my pre-assigned topic before Your Holiness. . . .

In the first place, therefore, I must touch upon the murky ignorance of these men [i.e., the flagellants], who are called, *people*. For as experience, the mistress of all things, teaches, the people are generally unlearned and crude, blinded by murky ignorance. . . . And in turn, most holy father, no learned men and also very few of the more esteemed laymen of vigorous intellect adhere to this sect, but they are nearly all common men. Even though some priests or friars follow or favor them, celebrating [divine services] in their presence as they journey along the

---

September 1349, but it is doubtful that this information would have reached Fayt in time for his sermon.

²Peter of Blois was a twelfth-century cleric who was famous for his corpus of Latin letters.

road, nevertheless they are not learned men, but crowned asses, ignorant of God's law, who follow them not for the sake of God, since they
are not devout men, but for the sake of alms and food. For instance, a
certain friar was interrogated in my presence and in that of many others, as to why he adhered to them, when he heard and knew that their
deeds and rites were displeasing to the bishops and greater clerics. He
answered: "Surely, we need to live off the goods of the burgesses of this
town [who support the flagellants], and no matter whether it be good or
bad what they do, we must defer to them [so that we can eat]." Therefore, except for such priests and friars, nearly all the other [flagellants]
are common men and, as a consequence, are unlearned, ignorant, and
crude. Moreover, this lack of learning and ignorance is the reason why
many of them believe that this sect is holy and licit. For they see certain
signs giving the appearance of goodness, but they do not know how to
truly discern between good and evil. . . .

In this way, these simple and ignorant people, deceived as if caught in
snares, believe that this sect is holy and licit, indeed to such an extent,
that they also believe that by their penance [i.e., flagellation], they
obtain a full remission of sins, reckoning that this is equivalent to a pilgrimage to Rome during a jubilee year. They also believe that these Flagellants can work miracles through the holiness of their penance. For
example, I have seen sick people brought before the Flagellants in order
that they might get their health back, and the Flagellants would lay their
caps and whips upon the sick so that they might get well. Indeed, some
simple people have become so deluded in this regard, that they venerate
the blood that they shed during their whipping as [holy] relics. Thus,
I have seen in a certain town how, as they whipped themselves and a
little blood ran down their backs, some old ladies and other simple folk
wiped up the blood with pieces of linen cloth, and they applied these to
their eyes and to the eyes of others like relics. And this the miserable
Flagellants allow to be done in order to make for a great spectacle. But,
as I have said, the reason for these abuses was, for the most part, their
murky ignorance. . . .

Secondly, I must touch upon a theme I mentioned already with regard
to these Flagellants: that is, their number, [or] copious quantity, as when
I said, "throughout all the provinces, etc." Literally, most holy father, the
multitude of such men is so great that there is hardly any great province
of Christendom to which this sect has not come. For it is said that they
had their origins in Germany under a certain religious man, and from
there they passed through the borders of Hungary, Bohemia, and many

other Eastern regions.[3] They also traveled north, into Frisia, Brabant, Hanover, Flanders, and the lower part of France, namely, into Picardy.[4] Indeed, I can say in brief that these people have now spread to the east, south, west, and north. . . . And this is one reason why princes and prelates, until now, have not proceeded to properly punish [the flagellants], because sometimes penalties have been set aside or deferred due to the sheer multitude of delinquents. . . . Also, they saw that this multitude [of flagellants] was so great, and their power was such that, even if they wished to proceed against them, they in turn would wish to resist [the actions taken against them]. This they have already done in several regions, such as in Bohemia, where they killed priests and clerics, towards whom the laity were completely hostile, as has been true since ancient times, [and] from this even worse things might follow, such as rebellions against princes and schisms against the Church. . . .

Thirdly, I must touch upon something I have already mentioned: their curious vanity, insofar as this affects us, as when I said that "they make use of new rules and ceremonies." This relates to a certain vanity and curiosity of the soul, but without the great need for, or evident usefulness in, changing ancient laws and observances nor in introducing new ones. For this is dangerous and harmful to the public weal. . . . But if one asks, what are the rules, ceremonies, or observances that the Flagellants follow, I answer that these are so many that I would not know how to explain them all. Nevertheless, out of them all, I can recall thirteen observances that they adhere to by virtue of their statutes and rules:

1) They possess five things to mark them off from all others, as did the divisive Pharisees, namely: a linen garment, running from the loins down to their feet, which they wear only at certain times [i.e., when they perform their whipping ceremonies]; a [walking] stick or staff; a cloak, on which the staff is depicted both in front and behind; a cap; and a whip, from which hang 3 or 4 leather thongs or rope cords, having at the ends knots with steel points in them.

---

[3]Another contemporary Flemish observer of the flagellants, Boendale of Brabant, states that the flagellants originally came out of Austria and Hungary, while the sermon in the flagellant scroll excerpted in Document 22 attributes their origins to a group of seven flagellants who arose in Jerusalem and then "came into the land of Hungary," and from there spread westward.

[4]There is little supporting evidence that the flagellants entered southern France. The French continuation of the chronicle of Guillaume de Nangis, for example, states that the flagellants "did not come to Paris nor to the French regions prohibited to them by the king of France." A party of one hundred flagellants from Basel allegedly entered Avignon, but they were immediately suppressed by Pope Clement VI.

2) Many, having gathered together from one town, then travel through other towns for thirty days, carrying [before them] crosses and banners.

3) They fast every Friday, asserting that to not fast on Friday is a sin for every Christian.

4) Twice a day they whip themselves in a public place with the afore-mentioned whips on their naked bodies from the loins upwards; also, at certain times [in the ceremony] they prostrate themselves down to the ground.

5) During this whipping they pierce themselves to the point of shedding blood, reckoning that this pleases God, like the priests of Baal. . . .

6) As they whip themselves in the market square and other public places, arranged in a ring like in a ring dance, they have three or four lead singers among them, who sing verse by verse certain songs, which they have composed on the subject of their penance, with the whole congregation singing each verse back in response.

7) If a woman enters their ring as they are performing their penance [i.e., whipping], they consider their penance to have been profaned and they start over from the beginning.

8) If it happens that they stay in a town for several days, it becomes necessary that each of them change hosts every day, not recollecting the word of Christ in Matthew 10:[11]: "In whatever city or town you shall enter, enquire who in it is worthy, and there abide until you go thence." . . .

9) Upon greeting honest persons, they do not doff their caps; indeed, what is worse, they do not take off the caps from their heads even when the body of Christ is elevated [in church during the Mass].

10) When they are at the dinner-table, they cannot eat bread unless the bread is broken by another.

11) In washing their hands, they cannot have water poured over their hands, but only when the basin is placed before them on the ground, do they dip their hands into the water.

12) For 30 days, they must do their penance, [and] they must stay away from their wives, even though their consent [to this] has not been asked for; yet the apostle [Paul] said in 1 Corinthians 7:[5]: "Defraud not one another, except, perhaps, by consent, for a time, that you may give yourself to prayer."

13) Everywhere [they go] they strive to kill the Jews, reckoning that they please God by exterminating the Jews, not heeding Psalm 58:[12]: "God shall let me see over my enemies; slay them not.". . . [Fayt marshals other, similar arguments in defense of the Jews by St. Augustine

of Hippo and St. Bernard of Clairvaux.] If the aforesaid Flagellants were to diligently heed such [arguments], they would not reckon themselves to be pleasing God by exterminating the Jews. But it is true that there is only one reason why they wish to kill them: They accuse them of being the cause of this great mortality, which began three years ago now and more [i.e., in 1346], and which still flourishes in several regions. For they say that they infected the water—upon which the vast majority of humanity depends for its nourishment—by throwing poison into springs and wells. Nor do they wish to believe that the epidemic, that is, the infection of the air caused by heavenly bodies [i.e., the planets], was the reason behind the aforesaid mortality, even though astronomers predicted a long time beforehand that this would happen based on [their reading of] the course of the stars.[5]

These and many other unsuitable observances they perform and follow in accordance with their statutes and rules. . . . Therefore, as you know full well, it would be least advantageous for your realm, namely, the Church militant, if this sect [of the flagellants] were to grow any further by means of the pretense that you seem to approve of them by keeping silent in this regard. In the name of my aforesaid lords [i.e., the masters of theology of Paris], whose messenger I am, although unworthy, I humbly beseech Your Holiness, on bended knee from [the depths] of my heart, that you see fit to eradicate this sect, or rather, this manifest error, so that this weed not choke off the wheat. . . .

[5]While it is true that the Jews were killed in many towns based on the accusation that they poisoned wells in order to infect Christians with plague, as we will see in the next section, there is little support for the idea that the flagellants were directly involved in the Jewish pogroms. Indeed, in some cases, the timing of these two events makes any sort of connection impossible: At Strasbourg and Constance, for example, the Jews were burned in February and early March of 1349, yet the flagellants did not arrive in these towns until June or July later that year.

THE POISON CONSPIRACY

During the first outbreak of the Black Death in 1348–1350, Jewish communities throughout much of Europe were accused of having poisoned drinking wells and springs and by this means of having spread the plague to Christians. On these grounds, Jews were then put to death in the thousands, giving rise to the term "Jewish pogroms" to refer to this event. Yet it is possible that the accusations of well poisoning during the Black Death were about more than anti-Judaism. At the very beginning of what I like to call the "poison conspiracy," it was "poor men and beggars of diverse nations" who were tried and executed on a charge of poisoning water and food in several towns in southern France (Document 25). Even when Jews did bear the brunt of the accusations, Christians were often listed as their accomplices. Meanwhile, the collection of letters from the town archives of Strasbourg provides a fascinating window into how the poison conspiracy spread from town to town across Europe via rumor and word of mouth (Document 26).

Traditionally, scholars of Jewish history have viewed the pogroms during the Black Death as marking a watershed in Christian-Jewish relations in Europe.[3] But the poison conspiracy had little to do with religiously based biases against Jews, such as informed the infamous "blood libels" (that is, accusations that Jews kidnapped and murdered Christian children in order to use their blood in Passover ceremonies). While Jews were a natural target of the poison conspiracy because of their presumed hostility toward Christians, almost anyone could be accused of being a poisoner, as the Dominican friar Henry Suso testifies in his autobiography.[4] Rather, the poison conspiracy was born out of an entirely rational explanation of the Black Death, namely, the "poison thesis" developed by plague doctors such as Gentile da Foligno (Document 9). Similarly, the poison conspiracy died out when its rational basis was undermined, namely, when people continued to die of plague long after all the Jews had been killed, as Konrad of Megenberg points out in the Jews' defense (Document 27).[5]

NOTES

[1] Richard Kieckhefer, "Radical Tendencies in the Flagellant Movement of the Mid-Fourteenth Century," *Journal of Medieval and Renaissance Studies* 4 (1974): 160–63. Kieckhefer debunks these notions, but they still persist in the popular image of the flagellants. For a detailed study of the emergence of a flagellant heretical sect in Thuringia after the movement of 1348–1349, see Ingrid Würth, *Geißler in Thüringen: Die Entstehung einter spätmittelalterlichen Häresie* (Berlin: Akademie Verlag, 2012).

[2] Kieckhefer, "Radical Tendencies," 163–65; Martin Erbstösser, *Sozialreligiöse Strömungen im Späten Mittelalter: Geissler, Freigeister und Waldenser im 14. Jahrhundert* (Berlin: Akademie Verlag, 1970), 10–69.

[3] Anna Foa, *The Jews of Europe after the Black Death*, trans. A. Grover (Berkeley: University of California Press, 2000), 13–16.

[4] Rosemary Horrox, trans. and ed., *The Black Death* (Manchester: Manchester University Press, 1994), 223–26.

[5] Samuel K. Cohn Jr., *The Black Death Transformed: Disease and Culture in Early Renaissance Europe* (London and New York: Arnold and Oxford University Press, 2003), 232. The only later outbreak of plague that sparked a massacre of Jews was in Krakow in 1360, where the disease struck for the first time.

25

ANDRÉ BENEDICT

Letter to the Jurors of Gerona
April 17, 1348

In the spring, perhaps in late March or early April, of 1348, the leading citizens, or "jurors," of the town of Gerona in Catalonia, near the coast of northeastern Spain just over the border from southern France, had written a letter to their counterparts in the town of Narbonne in Languedoc. The Geronan jurors had obviously heard of the plague's arrival in Narbonne, which was recorded there as early as March 1, and of the town's prosecution of those held responsible for the epidemic. Narbonne's de facto ruler, André Benedict, who was the vicar, or representative, for the town's lord, the Viscount Aymeric, wrote back on April 17, detailing the events of the past few weeks. Gerona itself was to be struck by plague later that spring, where it was recognized around May 1.

To the honorable, prudent, and discreet men, the jurors of the city of Gerona, André Benedict, vicar of the town of Narbonne [and] sheriff of the court of the distinguished and powerful man, the Lord Aymeric, by the grace of God viscount and lord of Narbonne, greetings, with every increase of prosperity. We have received your letters, containing how, as men who are prudent and wish to avoid future dangers, you desired to be informed by us by letter concerning the mortality of people which, by the grace of God, began to arise in Romania [i.e., Byzantium] and has [now] spread to parts of Avignon, Narbonne, and Carcassonne, [and] whether this happened due to potions or poisons[1] put in diverse parts by several people, whether this happened from some other cause, and if

---

[1]The Occitan word used here for poisons, *metzinis*, has a probable root in the Latin word *medicina*. This seems to confirm Benedict's familiarity with medical theories about plague, or at least with doctors' explanation of it, which is made even more clear at the end of the letter.

Christian Guilleré, "La Peste Noire à Gérone (1348)," *Annals de l'Institut d'Estudis Gironins* 27 (1984): 141–42.

anyone has been arrested for the aforesaid and confessed and if a punishment then followed and what kind and at whose instigation the said deeds are said to have been done.

Concerning [all of] which we notify you by the tenor of these presents that in Narbonne, in Carcassonne, and in the town of Grasse and neighboring regions there was and is so great a mortality of people throughout the whole of Lent [i.e., March 1 through April 11] and it has still not yet ceased, that a quarter of the inhabitants have been killed, according to common opinion. And many reeking of the crime of [spreading] the said potions and poison were discovered and arrested in Narbonne and elsewhere, [being] poor men and beggars of diverse nations carrying, as they [themselves] said and were seen [to have done], powdered poisons which they put in the water, houses, churches and foodstuffs in order to kill people. And in this way some freely confessed, but some [confessed] on pain of torture. And they persevered in their confessions, and they confessed that they had received these [poisons] in diverse places from certain persons, whose names they say they do not know. But [they say] that they were given money to induce them to spread the deadly poisons, nevertheless in truth an opinion is expressed that these things were done on behalf of enemies of the kingdom of France, although complete certainty cannot yet be had in this regard. Nevertheless, it is true that those who confessed were torn apart by red-hot iron pincers, were [then] quartered [disemboweled?], their hands cut off, and then they were burned. Justice was done against four of them in Narbonne, five in Carcassonne, [and] two in the town of Grasse, and many others were arrested for the aforesaid [crimes].

And even though some still assert natural [causes], that this [mortality] came from the two planets now reigning, we believe it is certain that the planets and poisons occur at the same time and induce the said mortalities. You should know that infirmities that come from the aforesaid [causes] are contagious, since once there is one dead person in any home, [then] the servants, family members, and parents are afflicted in that same way and from the same disease, and within three or four days all die. May the Most High in his mercy deign to deliver you and us from the aforesaid. We write you of the aforesaid with a very heavy heart, and we are prepared to please you in this and in weightier matters as true friends, and we can inform you more fully [of these things] as soon as we can. Given at Narbonne, on the 17th day of April, in the year of our Lord 1348.

26

Replies to Strasbourg's Interrogatory about the Jews
November 1348–January 1349

Sometime in the autumn of 1348, the mayor and town council of Stras-
bourg, having heard about proceedings against Jews in the Savoy, Swit-
zerland, and in the German kingdom, wrote to several towns in these
regions requesting information to help them decide what to do about their
own Jews. Twelve replies, some written in Latin and some in German,
survive in the town archives of Strasbourg. The longest and best known of
them all is the reply from the castellan of Chillon in the county of Savoy,
which details the interrogation of nine Jews and one Jewess on the charge
of poisoning local springs. But it is important to read and consider all
of the replies to be able to understand the complexity of the Christian
response to the Black Death. Only in this way can we gain a clear under-
standing of how information was conveyed and shared among various
communities, and thus how the poison conspiracy was born. We print the
letters here in the order in which they appear in the town archives, which
seems to be organized by date.

Lausanne [canton of Vaud, Switzerland], November 15, 1348 [Let-
ter in Latin]: *Sir Rudolf of Oron, lord of Artales and bailiff of Lausanne,*
and Michael of Vevey, esq., sautier *[i.e., official] of Lausanne, to Conrad*
of Winterthur, burghermeister of Strasbourg, and to the city councilors of
Strasbourg.

We have warmly received your gracious letters in this regard. In reply,
we send you the transcript of the confession[1] that was made by a certain
Jew, Bona Dies [literally, "Good Day"] by name, under our seal. This Jew

---

[1]The transcript of this confession does not survive, but it is likely to have been similar to those extracted from the Jews interrogated at Chillon and Châtel in the county of
Savoy, as related below.

Urkunden und Akten der Stadt Strassburg, ed. Wilhelm Wiegand et al., 15 vols. (Stras-
bourg: K. J. Trübner, 1879–1933), 5:164–79; *Recueil des Chroniques de Flandre*, ed. Joseph
Jean de Smet, 4 vols. (Brussels, 1837–1865), 2:344; *Fontes Rerum Germanicarum*, ed.
Johann Friedrich Böhmer, 4 vols. (Stuttgart: J. G. Cotta'scher Verlag, 1843–1868), 4:70.

was placed upon the wheel,[2] where he survived for four days and four nights, [and] for as long as he could speak, he persevered in what he first said without any change. And we have [already] informed you that, within the lordship of the count of Savoy, many Jews and also Christians have confessed to committing the same deeds and enormities [i.e., well poisoning]. For this reason, they were lawfully condemned and burned in that lordship. And know that some time ago we sent word of the confession made by the aforementioned Jew [Bona Dies] to our well-loved [colleagues], the officials and councilors of Bern [Switzerland] and Fribourg [Switzerland], at their request. Farewell. . . .

Bern [Switzerland], November 1348 [Letter in German]: *The schultheiz [i.e., mayor], council, and burghers of Bern to the burghermeister and council of the town of Strasbourg.*

As you wrote to us regarding the Jews [and] whether we had heard more about them and their poison, and in order to share the information [we have], this is to let you know that we sent to Solothurn [Switzerland] with an official complaint about the Jews and their murders, in order that they be judged. And a Jew [there], as he was being cut to pieces, stated that he was present [at the poisoning] and that the Jew, Köppli, and the Jew, Kürsenner, introduced poison into the fountain at Solothurn. He also told others to put poison into the wells, but whether this actually took place or not, he does not know. However, another Jew, as he was thrown in [to the fire], and as the heat began to rise, called out and said in public very loudly to all present: "You must know that all Jews in all countries know about the poison!"

Cologne [Lower Rhine, Germany], December 19, 1348 [Letter in Latin]: *The city of Cologne to the justices, officials, and councilors of the city of Strasbourg.*

Dear friends, Brother Henry, commendator of the [Dominican?] house of Cologne, who at one time resided in your city, related to us that he understood from some members of your council that the councilors of the town of Bern sent to you a certain Jewish prisoner, who was to inform you about the poisoning, and spreading of poison, from which Christians have died in various parts of the world. We are struggling [to make sense]

---

[2]The wheel, sometimes also known as the breaking wheel, was a form of torture and execution used in Germany up to the nineteenth century. Typically, the accused was tied onto the spokes of the wheel and then had his limbs broken by being beaten with a rod or club. The victim then died slowly of internal injuries.

of various rumors, but which is telling the truth, we do not know. And because it would be regrettable to pass over such a wicked crime, whose perpetrators are commonly said to be the Jews, without [obtaining] correct information, we therefore ask, by virtue of every mark of affection and good-will we can muster from your friendship, and in consideration of how much we reciprocate [such feelings], that you see fit to send back to us in writing, through the bearer of this letter, every bit of news that was mentioned and revealed by the said Jew, along with all of its circumstances, insofar as this is known, or can be known, to you. This is so that we may be able to legislate concerning, and take precautions against, such a poisoning in terms of a proportionate, foresighted response. Farewell. . . .

Zofingen [canton of Aargau, Switzerland], December 23, 1348 [Letter in German]: *The* schultheisz *[i.e., mayor] and council of Zofingen to the burghermeister and council of Strasbourg.*

As you wrote to us requesting that we send you the poison [that we found], we have to inform you that we are bound not to send the poison to anyone, since we have told and promised [not to do so] to all towns. But we can tell you that we found the poison under lock and key of our Jews. We also inform you that we made a trial of the poison on a dog, a pig, and a chicken, with the result that they [all] died of the poison, and we inform you that we put three Jews and a [Christian?] woman on the wheel, in accordance with proper procedure and information, as your messenger witnessed. The other Jews that we still have in custody are imprisoned, as required by law, and because [they are awaiting trial] by our procurators. You should also know that we can say under oath that the above facts are all true. If you do not believe these things as we have described, please send us one, two, or three whom you trust, [and] we will let them see the poison and make a trial of it as we have done before many honorable men. . . .

Colmar [Alsace, German kingdom], December 29, 1348 [Letter in German]: *The burghermeister and council of Colmar, to the burghermeister and council of the town of Strasbourg.*

This is to inform you that on Saturday night [December 27], we questioned, owing to the unrest, one of our Jews named Heggman, who is currently afoot and incites the Jews and who was known beforehand to be dishonest. He said during questioning, and also later, that Master Jacob "the Burner," a Jew residing in your parts, sent him some time ago a letter and some poison, and that he asked in the letter that he put the poison into the wells at Colmar. And [he said] that about four weeks ago he put the poison into a well that is outside our town, near the open road that goes up the valley towards Keysersberg [Alsace]. And [he said] that he promised to give his mother-in-law, Belin, a Jewess, ten pounds if she would put poison in the wells, and that about four weeks ago she did put poison in the nearest well to Ammerschwihr [Alsace].[3] And also, this Jewess [Belin] confessed that she did all this. You should also know that we found in the house of the same Jew [Heggman] a seal cut in soap that was made from the seal of Endingen [am Kaiserstuhl, Upper Rhine, Germany],[4] and we also found a letter on him, sealed with the same seal, and we sent to Endingen to request that the Jew and Jewess be punished according to the law. . . .

Münsingen [canton of Bern, Switzerland], undated, but probably end of 1348 [Letter in German]: *Sir Burkart "the Herdsman" of Münsingen, to the burghermeister of Strasbourg.*

As you bid me [tell you], and wrote to me, about the two baptized Jews that I allegedly executed, you should know that I executed them both, and they both publicly and in court stated that they carried poison and poisoned several wells. You should also know that one of them warned us and said that no Jew cared so much as about three things: first, how they can debase pennies [i.e., money]; second, how to ruin Christianity; third, that as they eke out an existence, none of their children beyond the age of four becomes a good Christian. And he stated publicly in front of me and two [other] witnesses, that he and his wife claimed to be Christians for about three years, but that they never believed in Christ. Then I asked him and his wife and the other one, whether they wished to die in the Christian faith. They stated publicly in front of me and the others that they wished to die in the Jewish faith. You should also know that when they were put on the wheel, [they confessed] that most of the poison they have now came from the Jews of Mainz, in particular from one whose name I cannot write to you now, but who sold some mixtures containing the poison. You should also know that he asked me to warn Christendom that no one should trust a baptized Jew. So I warn you, in good faith, that you should beware of them.

[3]All these towns are located within a close radius of each other in the Alsace region. Keysersberg is seven miles southeast of Colmar, while Ammerschwihr is five and a half miles northwest of Colmar. Colmar is about forty-five miles due south of Strasbourg.
    [4]It is not clear whether this is Endingen am Kaiserstuhl, which is twenty-two miles due east of Colmar in Germany, or Endingen in Switzerland, which is nearly eighty miles away to the south and east, but which was known for having a large Jewish community.

Chillon [canton of Vaud, Switzerland], undated, but probably end of 1348 [Letter in Latin]: *Castellan of Chillon, to the official, councilors, and community of the city of Strasbourg.*

Since I understand that you desire to know the confessions of the Jews and the proofs found against them, you should be aware that the people of Bern have made a copy of the interrogations and confessions of the Jews newly residing in their parts, who were accused of putting poison into wells and many other places, and that what is contained in this copy is absolutely true. And many Jews, because they confessed after being put to the question [i.e., tortured], and some confessed without torture, were put on trial and sentenced to be burnt. Also some Christians, to whom some Jews had entrusted their poison in order to kill Christians, were placed on the wheel and tortured. For the burning of the Jews and the torture of the said Christians has been done in many places in the county of Savoy. May the Almighty preserve you.

Here follows the confession of the Jews of Villeneuve [canton of Vaud, Switzerland] made on September 15 in the year of our Lord 1348 in the castle of Chillon, where they were detained, who were accused of putting poison into wells, cisterns, and other places, as well as into food, in order to kill and destroy the entire Christian religion.

Balavigny, a Jewish surgeon living at Thonon[-les-Bains, county of Savoy], was nonetheless imprisoned at Chillon because he was apprehended within the castellan's jurisdiction. He was briefly put to the question, and when he was released from the torture, he confessed after a long interval of time that around ten weeks ago, Rabbi Jacob, who had come from Toledo [Spain] and was staying at Chambéry [county of Savoy] since Easter [April 20], sent to him at Thonon through a certain Jewish serving boy a heap of poison about the size of an egg, which was in the form of a powder enclosed in a sack of fine, sewn leather, together with a certain letter, in which he ordered him under pain of excommunication and out of obedience to his religion to put the said poison into the greatest and most public well of the town, which was used the most often, in order to poison the people who would use the water of this well. And he was not to reveal this to anyone at all under the aforesaid penalty. It also was stated in the said letter that similar things were ordered in other mandates sent out by the Jewish rabbis of his religion to diverse and various places.

And he confessed that late one evening he put the said quantity of poison or powder under a stone in the spring by the lake-shore of Thonon. He also confessed that the said serving boy showed him many letters commanding the said deed or poisoning which were addressed to many other Jews: Some were directed in particular to Mossoiet, Banditon, and Samolet at Villeneuve; some to Musseo, Abraham, and Aquetus of Montreux [canton of Vaud, Switzerland], Jews at La Tour de Vevey [canton of Vaud, Switzerland]; some to Beneton of St. Maurice [canton of Valais, Switzerland] and to his son; and some directed to Vivian, Jacob, Aquetus, and Sonetus, Jews at Évian[-les-Bains, county of Savoy]; also, some to Hebrea and Musset, Jews at Monthey [canton of Valais, Switzerland]. And the said serving boy told him that he carried many other letters to various and remote places, but he does not know to whom they were addressed. Also, he confessed that after he put the said poison in the spring of Thonon, he expressly forbade his wife and children from using that spring but refused to tell them why. In the presence of very many trustworthy witnesses, he confessed by the faith in his religion and in all that is contained in the five books of Moses [Pentateuch] that the aforementioned things were absolutely true.

Also, on the following day, Balavigny, of his own free will and without being put to the question, confirmed that his said confession was true, repeating it word for word, in the presence of very many trustworthy witnesses. What is more, he freely confessed that on the day when he came back from La Tour de Vevey, he threw into a spring below Montreux, namely, the spring *de la Conereyde*, a quantity of poison the size of a nut, wrapped in a rag, which had been given to him by Aquetus of Montreux who lived in La Tour. The location of this poison he told and revealed to Manssionnus, a Jew living in Villeneuve, and to Delosatz, son of Musselotus, so that they would not drink from that spring. Also, he described the said poison as being red and black in color.

Also, on September 19 Balavigny confessed, without being tortured, that three weeks after Pentecost [i.e., three weeks from June 8], Mussus, a Jew of Villenueve, told him that he had put poison in the *Bornellorum* fountain of Villenueve, located, namely, in *la douane* [customs house], and he told him that afterwards he did not drink from that water but from the lake. He also confesses that Mussus the Jew told him that he had likewise put poison in the *Bornellorum* fountain of Chillon, located, namely, in *la douane*, under some stones. The fountain was then investigated and the said poison was found, which was then given to a certain Jew, who died thereafter, proving that it was poison. He also says that the rabbis of his religion had commanded him and other Jews to abstain from drinking the water for nine straight days from the day of its being poisoned, and he says that as soon as he put the poison in its receptacle, as he related above, he warned other Jews.

He also confesses that a good two months ago he was at Évian, and he spoke with Jacob the Jew concerning this matter, and among other things he asked Jacob if he had a letter and poison like the others. Jacob answered that yes, he did. Afterwards he asked him if he did what he was commanded, to which Jacob answered that he had not planted the poison himself, but had given it to Savetus the Jew, who put it in the spring *de Morer* at Évian. He urged Balavigny to obey orders and carry through this business just as well as he did.

He confesses that Aquetus of Montreux told him that he had put poison in the spring above La Tour, which he uses from time to time when he is at La Tour. He confesses that Samolet told him that he had put poison which he had received into a certain spring, but would not describe to him the spring.

Also, Balavigny says that, speaking as a surgeon, when someone gets sick from the poison and someone else touches him when he is sweating from his illness, that someone else will quickly feel worse from that touch. Also, one can be infected by the breath of the sick. And he believes these things to be true, because he has heard them explained by expert physicians. And it is certain that other Jews cannot acquit themselves of this charge, since they are well aware and are guilty of the aforesaid practices.

Balavigny was taken in a boat across the lake from Chillon to Clarens [canton of Vaud, Switzerland] in order to look for and identify the spring in which he had put the poison, as he confessed. When, coming up from below, he arrived at the place and saw the spring where he had put the poison, he said: "Here is the spring where I put the poison." The spring was searched in his presence and a linen rag or cloth, in which the poison had been enclosed, was found at the outlet of a stream that issues from the spring, by the notary public, Henry Girard, with many persons present, and it was shown to the Jew. He confessed and confirmed that it was the linen rag or cloth in which he had wrapped the poison and which he had put in the public spring, adding that the poison has the appearance of two colors, black and red. The linen rag or cloth was taken away and is in safe keeping.

Also, Balavigny confesses that all and several of the above things are true, adding that he believes the poison to come from the basilisk,[5]

---

[5]A legendary kind of snake said to be so venomous that it could kill with a single glance.

because the aforementioned poison cannot act except with the basilisk's intervention, as he has heard tell, and he is certain this is the case. . . .

Summary of remaining confessions: On September 15 at Chillon, Banditon of Villeneuve and Mamson of Villeneuve both confessed, a day after being tortured, to poisoning springs on the orders of Rabbi Jacob of Toledo and of a Jew called Provenzal. Mamson added that, "none of the Jews can acquit themselves of the aforesaid charges, because all alike are aware and guilty of the above."

On October 8–18 at Chillon, the Jewess Belieta, wife of Aquetus of Villeneuve, confessed after torture that the Jew, Provenzal, gave her poison to put into springs. Aquetus of Villeneuve, son of Banditon, also confessed, after being accused by Aquetus, son of Belieta, to receiving poison from Provenzal. He added that the Jews of Villeneuve took counsel among themselves about the poisoning outside the upper gate, and that "the Jews well deserved death and that he had no wish to escape being put to death immediately, because he well deserved death."

On October 10 at the castle of Châtel (county of Savoy), Agimetus the Jew and Jocetus the Jew confessed after torture that they poisoned wells and springs on the orders of Rabbi Rubi Peyret of Chambéry and in return for payment or the promise of payment. Agimetus further confessed he poisoned wells and springs as far away as Venice, Calabria, Apulia, Barletta, and Toulouse, where he traveled on business for the trading house of Claus de Rances to buy silk. On the same day and place, Iconetus of Bas and Aquetus Rubi of Warembon confessed after torture to poisoning springs near Brussels, Mons, and Geneva after being paid to do so by Abuget, "the most powerful and richest Jew of Bas," and by Salmin the Jew. Aquetus added that he had done the poisoning because of his "love for pranks" (dilectio ludi), and that "he now repented of what he had done."

On October 11 at Châtel, Aquetus, son of Jocetus the Jew, confessed after torture that he poisoned a well at Chambéry on the orders of Rabbi Rubi Peyret.

Freiburg and Waldkirch [Upper Rhine, Germany], undated, but probably end of 1348 [Letter in German]: *Anonymous record of the interrogation of the Jews at Freiburg and Waldkirch.*

Let it be known that Meiger Nasse, a Jew of Freiburg, confessed that he placed a small bag, about a hand long, in the well of Freiburg. Then he was asked how he did this. He said: "Where the stones are piled and joined together, I broke out one of the stones and put the little bag inside and closed it up again, and I did this after Our Lady's Day [March 25], before I left for Basel." He also said that the Jews of Strasbourg, Basel, Breisach [about nineteen miles from Freiburg], and Freiburg all know well about the poison, and that the Jews of Breisach wanted to destroy the castle and the town, and that he was present when the wells in Breisach were poisoned. He also said that there were four Jews in Breisach with whom he took counsel on how to poison the wells. And he named the four Jews: Ulle Smeriande, Judeli, Schöbeli, and Vifelman, and these four had also sent out letters from Breisach [to order other poisonings], as they had told him.

Let it also be known that Gotlieb the Jew stated, without any torture, that he had poisoned a well in Waldkirch; he also identified the well, which is called *Buchenbühl*. And he told us at the same time that the Jews in Waldkirch had instructed him [to do this]. Then he was asked how he obtained the poison; he said, without any torture, that a Jew named Anselm of Veringen[-stadt, about eighty-five miles east of Waldkirch and Freiburg] had come across the sea from Jerusalem to Strasbourg, and also to Freiburg. And when he heard that [Anselm] had come to Freiburg, he went from Waldkirch to Freiburg so that he could meet Anselm. And when he met [Anselm], he asked after his sister, and then about the poison. Anselm told him that he had brought poison from across the sea, and that this same poison was prepared with the same materials [as here], [and] that one places it in a well. Whoever among the Jews then drank the water, would suffer no injury. But if Christians drank it, they would die in a short time or longer; it would work. Then he was also asked what he gave Anselm for the poison. He said: "I gave him nothing for it when I heard that our faith would be strengthened by it." He also said that Anselm told him that he had left the poison in Freiburg.

He also stated that more of the poison had been buried in Freiburg in the houses of the Jews. He further said that *Frau* Guthilt the Jewess had gone across the sea and that she brought back a box full of poison to Freiburg, and that she tried the poison but that it didn't work. He added that the Jews of Freiburg received a letter from the Jews of Avignon as to whether, at first, they would share the poison. He also said that [the Jew] Swendewin told him that he had poisoned the well in Freiburg, and that he and all the Jews of Freiburg used the well early in the morning, and that during the day he went to the well and poured all [the poison] out. He also said that if anyone died in the French country, this all happened because of the Jews.

Let it also be known that Jekeli Gotlieb, a Jew of Freiburg, stated that he and Manne the Jew, Jekeli von Kestenholtze, Meiger Friburg,

Meiger Nasse, Leblange Gumpeli, Bunscheli Gumpreht, son-in-law of the blind Jew Frumolt, Enseli, son-in-law of Davit Kuchen—all these Jews conspired in the house of Merkelin the Jew, and in other Jewish houses, to poison the well and other waters with the poison that they had, and to give him 40 pounds in order to poison the wells of the town. He didn't want to do it. After some time, a Jew from Strasbourg came, by the name of Swendewin. We agreed that he should poison the well and we gave him 26 guilders. The guilders were given to him by Manne, Jekeli of Kestenholtz[e], Meiger Friburg, and Leblange. And he said that the same Swendewin told him that he had placed the poison in the well, in a small leather pouch. He also said that the poison first came from Basel, and that it was sent by Anselm and Kopeli, who recommended that they all should become active and serious [about poisoning] in this land. He also said that they poisoned all the wells located between Freiburg, Breisach, and Endingen, and he said that it took about ten weeks for them to do it. And because of the conspiracy, they took [the poison] from one town to another, and all the Jews in Strasbourg, Basel, Breisach, and Freiburg know about it. And afterwards, the Jews promised him that they would do their best [to poison the wells] in the towns and surrounding [countryside]. Then the Jews gathered in a council as to what they should do with the poison, and they agreed that Meiger Nasse should take the poison and travel throughout the land with the poison, so that he could poison all the wells and waters. He made these statements without any torture, and he related the journeys that he was to undertake.

Liebkind [the Jew] said that all the Jews wanted to have [some] of the poison. He was asked why this was so. He answered that it was because so many Christians had killed Jews when "King Armleder"[6] was there.

This is what the Jews in Waldkirch did:

First, Vivelin [the Jew] told about the well at *Kelbenau*, into which he placed a rag with poison. In Weiler [near Rottenburg, southwest Germany], they dug up the well above the village and poured poison into it. Near the Sömmer Bridge, at the source [of the spring], they poured in poison [contained] in a rag, and in the lower village they placed it in the *Tetenbach* [well, contained] in a rag. Up near Barnloch [Bavaria, Germany], they placed it

---

[6]The Armleder massacres occurred in the Alsace region in 1338–1339, ten years before the Black Death. Led by an innkeeper named John Zimberlin, who was styled "King Armleder" after the leather straps tied around his arms, the Armleder band marauded through Alsace, killing many Jews, until pursued by imperial forces and the local nobility, who managed to suppress their activities for a time.

in the well [contained] in a rag. Also, in the forest, they placed it in the *Schuler* spring in a rag. They also [placed it] in the *Luten* well, near the Küchelin's house, [contained] in a rag. Also, [they placed it] in the *Buchenbühl* [well] in a rag. The well for the hospital is also poisoned. Also, the well in the courtyard of St. Martin's [church] was poisoned in a rag; this well was poisoned by Vivelin and Jacob. [Jekeli] Gotlieb and his worker put poison in the well of St. Peter-in-the-Fields. At Buchholz [Middle Rhine, Germany], *Sidenfadem's* well is poisoned; this was done by a foreign Jew.

Oberehnheim [or Obernai, Alsace], undated, but probably end of 1348 [Letter in German]: *The* schultheisz *[i.e., mayor] and council of Oberehnheim, to the burghermeister and council and "the Forty that have been selected because of the Jews" in the town of Strasbourg.*

We inform you that we arrested five of our Jews today, Monday, and questioned them because of poison, and they stated that seven of our wells in Oberehnheim are poisoned. And the eldest of them said that the poison was sent by the rich Jews, Jekelin and Aharam, who are resident here and who sent them to Oberehnheim, and that they had agreed to this in Speyer about half a year ago. The burghers of our council have heard this, and other honorable citizens informed us that they heard it [also]. We attest to this [by oath] sworn without any threats. . . .

Kenzingen [14 miles north of Freiburg, Upper Rhine, Germany], undated, but probably end of 1348 [Letter in German]: *Anonymous record of the interrogations of the Jews at Kenzingen.*

This is what the Jews in Kenzingen said: that they poisoned all the wells in Kenzingen, and the brook called the *Steinspalte* near the House of *Vortut* in old Kenzingen. Since then, poison was found in the same brook. Jacob [the Jew] stated in particular that he ritually killed two Christian children, one in Munich and one in Tübingen. Abraham [the Jew] had killed a [Christian] child about a year old in Strasbourg, who had been bought for 10 pounds and whatever sauerkraut they could find. They also poisoned and shat into the wine at the Keppenbach winery, belonging to Rudolf Schafner, and they also shat into the wine press. And they also shat into the [town] moat that became empty of fish and frogs that are [now] all dead. They told of all this, and that they also shat into the cistern at *Kürnberg*. And they mentioned the names of the most affluent Jews in Strasbourg, namely: Jacob "the Rich," Süskind, and Abraham, Jews of Strasbourg. There were present during these statements the following witnesses: the *schultheize* [i.e., the mayor]; [*Herr*] Brenner; [*Herr*] Zunde; [*Herr*] Rüber; Herman Zechlin; Berschi of Riegel; [*Herr*] Spiser; [*Herr*] Kilcherre; Johan and Cunze, brothers of [*Herr*] Keppenbach;

Henni Löser; Henni of Maltertingen; [*Herr*] Sigbott; Rudolf of Ringisheim. We affirm that we heard the aforementioned things, by the oath we swore here, and others who are not members of the council affirm these things, by the oath sworn to our Lord.

Breisach [Upper Rhine, Germany], undated, but probably end of 1348 [Letter in German]: *Burghermeister and council of Breisach, to the burghermeister and council of Strasbourg.*

We inform you that since the time when your good messengers were here, Paulus, a baptized Jew whom we had taken prisoner, stated, after he had been put on the wheel for three [days], [confessed] that, regarding the poison, the *Heigim* [i.e., leader] of the Jews, Löwelin of Marle, who resides in Sélestat [Alsace], gave two Jews 3,000 guilders as payment [for poisoning]. And one [of the Jews] was called Saul Hogge, and he is baptized now and he now resides in the *Haiwart* [street or district] across from the [public] bath, and he married a painter's daughter. The other one was called Salman Brüne, and he resides in the jugsmith's house in Jews' Alley and he married the armorer's daughter. And [Löwelin] also gave them a little bag [of poison] and told them to do with it as they would be instructed. The same [Saul] Hogge spoke to the aforementioned Paulus after Pentecost [i.e., June 8] as to whether he wanted to earn money, [but] he didn't want to. And the same [Saul] Hogge also sent a servant away, who was named Simmunt, who was a messenger for the Jews. And after [Paulus] had been baptized, he resided in the Horse Market, in a house called "the Moon," [and] he did not go back [to the Jewish Quarter]. The same Paulus also said that Johannes Vingot, who opened the [barrel] hoops in Köppelin's cellar and who now works as a plumber, said in front of the same Paulus, which was fourteen days before St. John [the Baptist's] Day [i.e., fourteen days before August 29], that he didn't know any man who was worse to Christendom than himself, and they all believed him. Then, three days later, [Johannes Vingot] came to him and asked him where the poison was. He didn't want to tell him, and the same [Johannes] Vingot went away and bought a penny's worth of material from a dealer, who sets up [shop] near the main church next to the grating near the back door, on the left hand side, and [Johannes Vingot] said that he wanted to kill the cats in his house with it. The same Paulus also said that the aforementioned *Hegim* of Sélestat [i.e., Löwelin of Marle] was coming to Strasbourg. [Paulus] also told me that his father pressured him very much to become a Jew again. He said all these things regarding the trip the [*Hegim*] was going to take [to Strasbourg] without fear [of torture] and voluntarily, [and] that he knew this to be so. For this reason, we have written it down for you, so that you can take measures in the future when your messenger brings this to you in due time.

Cologne, January 12, 1349 [Letter in Latin]: *The justices, officials, and councilors of the city of Cologne to the burghermeister, Conrad of Winterthur, and to the officials and councilors of the city of Strasbourg.*

Dearest friends, diverse and various rumors are now flying about on every side against Judaism and the Jews concerning this sudden and unforeseen mortality among the Christian faithful, which—oh woe!— has raged in various parts of the world and is still lamentably active in some places. And many-winged Fame is exerting herself in this way among you as well as us and among other towns, [alleging] that this mortality first arose, and still does so, by means of the poisoning of springs and wells, into which the Jews felt bound to scatter poisonous things. When it came to our attention that some accusations had been brought against the Jews in some small towns and villages, we sent letters containing our requests [for information] to you and to other cities and towns many times, in order that we might know the full truth about these rumors, and we faithfully and diligently conducted investigations ourselves into the circumstances of such [alleged] misdeeds. Yet we have still been unable to uncover the simple truth about the Jews, either from you or from others, and, based on what you have most recently written to us, you still do not know the truth about these things either.

For if a massacre of Jews were to be allowed in the major cities—which we are intent upon preventing in our city, insofar as we are able and for as long as we find [the Jews] blameless and innocent of these and similar misdeeds—many other scandals and disturbances could arise, and the common folk could, as a consequence, be inclined to instigate a popular uprising, which have given rise to much misery and devastation in the cities and towns where such uprisings occur. And because we still reckon that it is truer to say that the aforesaid mortality and its circumstances are a plague from God and nothing else, we are resolved to in no way allow the Jews of our city to be molested on account of such flying rumors, but, rather, like our predecessors, we intend to faithfully defend and protect them, and we are of the firm opinion that you should do the same. Therefore, out of friendship, we kindly and earnestly beseech you, knowing that you are circumspect in everything you do, to strive to proceed reasonably and discreetly in this business of the Jews, in accordance with the law and reason. In this way, you may anticipate, and thus avert, the popular uprisings from which massacres of the Jews and other disturbances could, not surprisingly, follow, and by your foresightedness, you may check the rage that the common folk feel towards the Jews and keep it from spreading down to the lower parts [of the Rhine], as it usually does. And you should strive to faithfully protect the Jews of your city and keep them safe, just as your predecessors defended them, until the truth [of the matter] is more fully known. For should such an uprising against the Jews occur among you, it is likely that this would also happen in other cities and towns, as has been seen [before]. Therefore, it would be best if you, as well as we and [all] the other major cities, proceed with foresight and caution in this business, since he who does not prudently plan for future events, frequently falls into unexpected dangers. Farewell, and should you have learned any definite news, either from kings and princes or from the Jews themselves, may it please you, insofar as this is convenient, to send this back to us in writing through the bearer of this letter.

Postscript: *According to the German chronicler Heinrich Truchsess of Diessenhofen, Cologne burnt its Jews on August 23, 1349, the same day as Mainz. The Flemish chronicler Gilles li Muisis provides this anecdote about what happened to the Jews of Cologne:*

But one should not neglect to mention what happened in the city of Cologne, which is a metropolis. In that city, there were a great number of Jews, and they had an assigned place [i.e., a ghetto] and they lived together as neighbors separate from Christians. And it happened that many Jews, fleeing from other places where they were put to death, came to Cologne, and they situated themselves there with other Jews. And there was [as a consequence] a great multitude of Jews there. But the citizens and inhabitants of the city, seeing this, held counsel [among themselves], like in other places, [and decided] that there was nothing to do but that they be destroyed. But the Jews armed themselves and sought out arms, along with those arms that they had in their possession as pledges from Christians, and they manfully resisted many times, nor were the citizens and others from the city able to vanquish them, because they hesitated to set fire to their houses, since the whole city could be destroyed. But it happened that the butchers and very many from the city sent false messages to the Jews saying that they would join with them, and on a certain day the Jews, being armed, attacked those from the city, and the Christians, knowing this, resisted, and there was a great battle there, but by the will of God the Jews were vanquished. And it is generally agreed that more than 25,000 of the Jews were slain; yet many of the Christians fell and died. And the place [ghetto] was destroyed and the dwellings and houses of the Jews were completely burnt; but the Christians had the victory.

27

KONRAD OF MEGENBERG

Concerning the Mortality in Germany

ca. 1350

Perhaps the most balanced and rational medieval author to comment on the pogroms against the Jews was the scholar and priest Konrad of Megenberg. In the following selection from his De Mortalitate in Alamannia *(Concerning the Mortality in Germany), he debates both sides of the question as to whether the Jews caused the plague through the poisoning of wells. Megenberg seems to have written this treatise in 1350.*

Therefore it is commonly believed in Germany that certain men called the Jews, who declare themselves to be bound by the Mosaic law and practice circumcision and who deny the crucified Christ and the true God made flesh from a pure virgin for the sins of human kind, poisoned the water of wells used for drinking and other human uses with a very potent poison; and that they did so throughout the various regions of the world where Christians and men of other faiths live with them, chiefly in order that, once the people of the Christian religion are dead, the kingdom of the Jewish race and their status as the Lord's anointed may be restored, which was taken away from them by the word of God, that is, by the only begotten flesh of God, as is written: "The scepter shall not be taken away," and again it says in Scripture: "until the Lord of Hosts shall come, etc."[1] And this belief is confirmed by the fact that in many wells

---

[1]The full passage from Genesis 49:10 reads: "The scepter shall not be taken away from Juda, nor a ruler from his thigh, till he come that is to be sent, and he shall be the expectation of nations."

Sabine Krüger, "Krise der Zeit als Ursache der Pest? Der Traktat *De mortalitate in Alamannia* des Konrad von Megenberg," in *Festschrift für Hermann Heimpel zum 70. Geburtstag am 19. September 1971* (Göttingen: Vandenhoeck and Ruprecht, 1971), 866–68.

and streams of Germany, little sacks have been found, which, so they say, are full of decay and brimming with the most deadly poison. This poison, so they affirm, was tested on brute animals, such as pigs, dogs, and chickens and other animals, by mixing it with something edible, namely bread or meat, so that in this way they would taste some of the vile poison. Immediately the animals succumbed to a most swift death and their life was snuffed out as in a moment.[2]

And again, [they cite the fact] that very many men, commonly called "sack-bearers" or "sack-porters" [i.e., vagabonds], have been apprehended, who, when put to various kinds of tortures, confessed to this crime and did not deny it, namely that they brought this deadly matter to the crowded places of the world in order to kill all Christian men throughout the land. And what is surprising is how many of these "sack-porters" or poisoners were Christians, who, while in the midst of an all-consuming fire, swore with their last breath that they were bribed by the Jews with money to commit this most wicked crime, that they were seduced into this evil by everything delectable in this world, nor could they restrain themselves in any way from their hearts' desire for these delights.

Therefore the Christian people throughout nearly the whole of Germany, moved by these reasons, rushed upon the Jewish race with fire and with a most violent fury stained their hands with their blood. And their nation perished, namely Hebrews of both sexes, at the hands of the Christians, so that neither the nursing infant nor the child enclosed in its mother's womb was spared. Oh, how much weeping and wailing and what fear of heart and hissing between teeth was to be seen among a forsaken people! You would have seen maidens and wives with an unforgettable look upon their angelic faces being slaughtered by stupid rustic men with axes and nailed clubs and other instruments of war without mercy, as if they were slaughtering pigs or strangling chickens that were destined for the kitchen. Also, sometimes in some places they [the Jews] shut themselves up in a house with the doors barred and, after setting the house on fire, they died by their own hands by slitting the throats of their children, along with their own.[3] Oh, what a wicked and detestable crime by the parents, which is thus visited upon their children, so that justly "they say to the mountains: 'Come, cover us' and

---

[2]In principle, Megenberg was not opposed to the concept of poison spreading the plague, as he employs it when discussing whether earthquakes caused the Black Death.

[3]Except for setting the house on fire, this was how the Jews of Mainz committed *kiddush ha-Shem* during the First Crusade in May 1096, according to the chronicle of Solomon Bar Simson. Having the throat cut with a knife recalled Abraham's attempted sacrifice of Isaac.

'Blessed are the barren who have not given birth,'" concerning which He [Christ] spoke the truth to mothers when he was led miserably to be crucified for our sins: "Daughters of Jerusalem, weep not over me, but weep for yourselves and for your children."[4] For He knew what was to happen to them now and in times past.

But although the Jewish people are justly detested by us Christians in accordance with the fundamentals of the Catholic faith, which are proven not only by the words of the prophets, but are also confirmed by the most manifest miracles of God, which they [the Jews] stubbornly deny, nevertheless it does not seem to me that the said opinion concerning the cause of so general a mortality throughout the whole world, with all due respect to whomever is expressing it, can be totally and sufficiently maintained. My reasoning is as follows: It is well known that in most places where the Hebrew people had remained, they themselves had died in droves from the same exact cause of this common mortality, as in the city of Vienna in Austria and in the city of Ratisbon in Bavaria, as well as in castles and fortresses where they were concealed by certain Christian noblemen. But it is not likely that the same people who ardently desire to multiply themselves upon the land should with malice aforethought destroy themselves and others of the same faith. And again: After the wells and cisterns full of stagnant water have been purified, and even when the original source and complete origin of the gushing and flow has been secured and finally blocked off, the people, who never used other springs, died in great numbers. To which one also can add that if there had been such poison that could infect brute animals, as our adversaries say they have tested on them, then without doubt horses, cows, and sheep and livestock that drink the water ought to have been infected and died in great number like humans, which has not been seen. Nor is it probable, as is claimed, that livestock get their water more often from rivers, so that thus they cannot be infected from such things as wells and trickling streams, since the whole populace of Bavaria in the cities bordering on the Danube and other navigable rivers only use the water of these same rivers and most scrupulously avoid well water, and nevertheless they have died.

Moreover, even after all the Jews in many places have been killed and completely driven out for nearly two years prior, the Death now first

---

[4]This is a rather garbled version of Luke 23:28–30: "But Jesus turning to them, said: 'Daughters of Jerusalem, weep not over me; but weep for yourselves, and for your children. For behold, the days shall come, wherein they will say: Blessed are the barren, and the wombs that have not borne, and the paps that have not given suck. Then shall they begin to say to the mountains: Fall upon us; and to the hills: Cover us.'"

strikes these same places with a strong hand and powerfully conquers the men who remain there, as in the city of Nuremberg in Swabia and in the countryside roundabout. For this and similar reasons it does not seem to me that the pitiful Jewish race is the cause of this general mortality which has spread throughout almost the whole world.

7

Environmental Explanations
and Responses

The sheer magnitude of the Black Death epidemic, and the environmental catastrophe it represented (at least in terms of its impact upon humans), forced a radical rethinking of medieval attitudes toward the environment.[1] No longer did humans see nature, acting on behalf of God, simply as playing an adversarial role against humans when natural disasters struck; instead, humans saw themselves as having a part to play in their relationship with nature, one in which they now held some accountability for their own actions with respect to the natural world.[2] This could be on a moral, metaphysical plane, as imagined by Gabriele de Mussis (Document 28) or, more prosaically, in the form of human pollution that now had to be regulated and restrained if its effects were not to redound onto humans to cause them harm (Document 30).[3] And there were the environmental signs, such as vaporous colors in the sky or mice and other vermin issuing from holes in the ground, that plague doctors listed for their readers as what to watch for in their natural surroundings so that they might take appropriate precautions, such as fleeing from a region about to be infected by plague.[4] Finally, there was also an interest in providing more natural explanations of plague, such as Konrad of Megenberg's discussion of earthquakes (Document 29). Megenberg's treatise can be considered an extension of the great outpouring of natural histories in the thirteenth century, when a more harmonious or collaborative relationship between humans and nature was envisioned that obviously came to a crashing end with the Black Death.

Researchers in the still emerging field of medieval environmental history continue to debate how to approach the diverse sources available to them. One approach is to adopt the interaction model, in which all sources of environmental history, whether written or artifactual (i.e., archaeological or material), are assumed to be the product of the interaction between nature (the "natural sphere of causation") and human culture (the "cultural sphere of causation").[5] A complete separation of these two spheres is deemed the "traditional," or outdated, approach.[6] But adhering too closely to this interaction model has led some environmental historians astray, particularly with regard to adopting the arguments of plague denial, which have been disproven by paleomicrobiology (see the introduction).[7] Some observations made by medieval authors had no reality in the natural world, while some phenomena that did exist in nature left barely a trace in the written or artifactual record.[8] Perhaps the best approach to medieval environmental sources is to examine each one individually, on its own merits, and with a careful regard to its context.

NOTES

[1]John Aberth, *An Environmental History of the Middle Ages: The Crucible of Nature* (London: Routledge, 2013), 8–9.

[2]David Herlihy, "Attitudes toward the Environment in Medieval Society," in *Historical Ecology: Essays on Environment and Social Change*, ed. Lester J. Bilsky (Port Washington, N.Y.: Kennikat Press, 1980), 100–116.

[3]Dolly Jørgensen, "The Medieval Sense of Smell, Stench and Sanitation," in *Les Cinq Sens de la Ville du Moyen Âge à nos Jours*, ed. Robert Beck, Ulrike Krampl, and Emmanuelle Retaillaud-Bajac (Tours, France: Presses Universitaires François-Rabelais, 2013), 301–13.

[4]This topic is addressed in more detail in John Aberth, *Doctoring the Black Death: Europe's Late Medieval Medical Response to Epidemic Disease* (Lanham, Md.: Rowman and Littlefield, forthcoming).

[5]Marina Fischer-Kowalski and Helga Weisz, "Society as Hybrid between Material and Symbolic Realms: Towards a Theoretical Framework of Society-Nature Interaction," *Advances in Human Ecology* 8 (1999): 215–51; Richard C. Hoffmann, *An Environmental History of Medieval Europe* (Cambridge: Cambridge University Press, 2014), 7–15. Hoffmann illustrates the interaction model concept with the aid of a Venn diagram.

[6]Hoffmann, *Environmental History*, 7. The only sources that Hoffmann excludes from the intersection area of his Venn diagram are "paleoscientific data," such as "inferences from tree rings, ice cores, isotopic analysis of organic items, animal bones," and other such "proxy data," which he places entirely in the nature portion of his diagram. Presumably, paleomicrobiological data identifying the *Yersinia pestis* bacterium in plague victims would also fall exclusively under the nature category.

[7]Ibid., 296. Hoffmann rejects the paleomicrobiological identification of the Black Death with plague on the grounds that, even when the DNA of a "particular pathogen," namely, *Yersinia pestis*, is found in a person buried in a mass grave pit, this still "is not definitive proof that the pathogen caused the individual's death, nor is it proof that the pathogen caused the epidemic associated with the pit." Yet the only way that *Yersinia pestis* DNA could have ended up in the dental pulp of a victim is by primary or secondary septicemia, which causes death 100 percent of the time.

[8]An example of the first assumption is Hoffmann's statement that medieval physicians were "well trained to observe symptoms" of disease and that their "detailed descriptions" accurately reflect patients' disease condition; in fact, however, many plague treatises simply recycle ancient diagnoses (e.g., that buboes can be red, yellow, or green, according to the *Prognostics* of Hippocrates). An example of the second assumption is Hoffmann's revisionist objections that rats are not mentioned by medieval writers during the Black Death and that they are not found among the bones and other artifacts recovered from archaeological sites. An absence of rats from the cultural or artifactual sphere, however, does not mean they were absent from nature: Rat bones require very fine sieving techniques for their archaeological recovery, while medieval observers were unlikely to observe sick or dying rats that burrowed deep underground or within existing structures to evade cannibalism from their own species. See Hoffmann, *Environmental History*, 14–15, 291, 294–95, 297.

28

GABRIELE DE MUSSIS

History of the Disease or Mortality of 1348
1348–1356

Gabriele de Mussis was a notary, or lawyer, from Piacenza in Italy. His account of the Black Death is perhaps best known for its description of the "biological warfare" waged by the Mongols in 1346, whereby they lobbed plague corpses into the town of Kaffa on the north coast of the Black Sea to spread the disease to the besieged Genoese inside. In this excerpt from the opening of Mussis's Historia de Morbo *(History of the Disease), the author imagines a dialogue between God and the Earth to explain the origins of the Black Death.*

May this stand as a perpetual reminder to everyone, now living and yet to be born, how almighty God, king of heaven, lord of the living and of the dead, who holds all things in his hand, looked down from on high and saw the entire human race slipping and sliding towards all kinds of wickedness, enmeshed in crimes, pursuing numberless transgressions, immersed up to their bowels in every kind of vice out of an unfathomable malice, bereft of all goodness, not fearing the judgments of God, and chasing after everything evil. No longer able to bear so many abominations, so many horrors, God called out to the Earth:

"What are you doing, Earth, held captive by gangs of worthless men, soiled with the filth of sinners? Are you totally helpless? What are you doing? Why do you not demand human blood in vengeance for this wrongdoing? Why do you tolerate my enemies and adversaries? When confronted by such wantonness, you ought to have already swallowed my opponents. Make yourself ready to exercise the vengeance which lies within your power."

"And I, the Earth, having been established at your command, will open my veins and swallow up an infinite number of criminals once you give the order. I will deny the usual fruits of the earth, I will not bring forth grain, wine, and oil."

A. W. Henschel, "Document zur Geschichte des Schwarzen todes," in *Archiv für die gesammte Medicin*, ed. Heinrich Haeser, 10 vols. (Jena: Mauke, 1841–1849), 2:45–46.

And when the very irate Judge gave the word, with thunder sent down from the heavens, He marshaled the elements, the planets, the stars, and the orders of the angels against the human race with an unspeakable judgment, and He armed every single animate being in order to exterminate the sinners, and He called them forth to execute His justice with quite a cruel stroke.

29

KONRAD OF MEGENBERG

Concerning the Mortality in Germany

ca. 1350

Possessing a great interest in the natural world, the German scholar and priest Konrad of Megenberg wrote the first book on natural history in the German language, the Book of Nature, *which was modeled on Thomas of Cantimpré's* On the Nature of Things, *although Megenberg adds many of his own observations. In this excerpt from* Concerning the Mortality in Germany, *Megenberg debates, in typical scholastic fashion, the merits of his preferred explanation for the Black Death, namely, earthquakes, against both self-raised objections to his position and alternative explanations, such as the wrath of God and planetary conjunctions. This section of Megenberg's treatise is also published separately under its own title,* Whether the mortality of these years proceeded from divine wrath on account of the iniquities of men, or from a certain natural course [of events]. *Although the authorship remains anonymous, a comparison with the original makes it clear that this was by Megenberg.*

Sabine Krüger, "Krise der Zeit als Ursache der Pest? Der Traktat *De mortalitate in Alamannia* des Konrad von Megenberg," *Festschrift für Hermann Heimpel zum 70. Geburtstag am 19. September 1971* (Göttingen: Vandenhoeck and Ruprecht, 1971), 864–82; Karl Sudhoff, "Pestschriften aus den ersten 150 Jahren nach der Epidemie des 'schwarzen Todes' 1348," *Archiv für Geschichte der Medizin* 11 (1919): 44–50.

First, it is argued that [the mortality] comes from divine wrath and indignation at the iniquities committed by men, because the aforesaid mortality ceases when God's anger and indignation is placated by men's prayers and devotions; therefore, it is by His anger and indignation that [the mortality] is inflicted [upon men]. . . . In opposition, it is argued that, while God may seem to have made this plague for the correction of men, experience teaches us that the people have in no way amended themselves of any vice, so that God would have done this [i.e., the plague] to no purpose, which is not to be admitted. Item, by this same reasoning, God would have struck down all mortal sinners, whereas we see that the opposite [is true].

Second, it is argued that [the mortality] comes from a certain natural course [of events], namely, by virtue of some constellation [i.e., conjunction of the planets], because the whole of the perceptible world is ruled by the motions of the heavenly bodies; therefore, it is from the heavens that this mortality is inflicted upon men. . . . In opposition, it is argued that no aspect or conjunction of the planets lasts for so long a time as this mortality has lasted, and still lasts; therefore, no celestial influence is a sufficient and immediate cause of the aforesaid mortality. The former statement is made clear by this, that among all the planets, only Saturn remains in each of the twelve houses [i.e., signs] for two and a half years, but it interrupts its stay in any of these due to the stations and retrogrades [i.e., backward movements] in its eccentric epicycle. For Saturn may travel through the entire zodiac in thirty years; therefore, it will stay in each of the twelve signs for two and a half years. But all the other planets run through their courses more briefly, which is why none of them can remain with [Saturn] in the same house for the full two and a half years. Moreover, it is clear that the oft-mentioned mortality lasts in various parts of the world for five or six years, nor is it finished yet; therefore this argument fails. . . . And once again, [I say] that immediately following an actual conjunction, there is a certain succession of time and causality, a definite order and regular progression in these matters. But it is clear that often the said mortality, from what I can gather, now moves towards the east and now in the opposite direction, and then changing direction leaps from the south to the north and retraces its steps in places already visited, in such a way as if it moves with an accidental or involuntary motion like some bodily form, which is propelled by winds in the airy regions. Surely, no version of the stars' properties has them revolve in this fashion. For this and similar reasons, it does not appear to me that this mortality came directly from the stars, but rather from an intermediate cause or many remote ones. . . .

Therefore, I put forward a fourth opinion, which I believe is more credible than the others, which is in line with the Hippocratic view of condition and location.[1] This is namely that the oft-mentioned mortality, as a product of the natural course [of events], is directly and intrinsically caused by a corrupt and poisonous exhalation from the earth, which infected the air in various parts of the world, and when breathed in by men suffocated them to the point of sudden extinction. In order to prove and clarify my position, I submit two arguments sufficiently grounded in natural science.

The first of these is that when air that is full of vapors and fumes is shut up and imprisoned for a long time in the earth, it becomes so corrupted in some corner of the earth that it may be turned into a potent poison to the human constitution. And [this is so] especially in caverns and the bowels of the earth, which cannot be ventilated by new and fresh air. This is proven by much experience taken from [cases of] wells that have lain unused for a long time and had their openings sealed for many years. For when such wells are opened and ought to be cleaned out, it not infrequently happens that the first man to go in is immediately suffocated, and sometimes many who follow him in turn.[2]

The second argument is that an earthquake is caused by an exhalation of the earth's fumes shut up in the bowels of the earth, which, when they forcefully batter the sides of the earth and cannot escape, they shake and move the earth. This cause of earthquakes is proven by all the philosophers of natural science, nor is it necessary to adduce the philosophers' reasoning in this regard. For I say, that a great vapor and corrupt air issued forth during a very great earthquake, which happened on St. Paul's day in the year of our Lord 1347 [January 25, 1348].[3] And like-

---

[1]This probably refers to the ancient work titled *Airs, Waters, and Places*, attributed to Hippocrates of Cos (460–377 BCE), which taught that an understanding of natural environments would enable one to diagnose diseases likely to strike a given location.

[2]Megenberg cites in support of this contention a contemporary incident occurring in the city of Ratisbon in his native Bavaria, "where upon opening a certain well unused for many years, three men died after entering it." The common "ignorant" folk attributed the deaths to a basilisk and had the well blocked up again.

[3]In his *Book of Nature*, Megenberg also mentions this famous earthquake, which is often referred to as the Friuli earthquake of 1348 (to distinguish it from the more recent one in 1976), named after its believed epicenter in the Friuli region of northeast Italy, near the border with Austria. The earthquake not only affected the town of Villach in Carinthia, which was buried under a landslide from the nearby slopes of Mt. Dobratsch, but also badly damaged the castle and cathedral in Udine in northeast Italy, and was felt as far away as Rome. Megenberg provides a more detailed explanation of earthquakes in chapter 33 of Book 2 of his *Book of Nature*, including what signs to look for when they are about to happen. See Konrad von Megenberg, *Buch der Natur, vol. 2: Critical Text*, ed. Robert Luff and George Steer (Tübingen: Max Niemeyer Verlag, 2003), 131–33.

wise, corrupt air from enclosed places in the earth, which was released in the course of other earthquakes and eruptions in the earth that happened later, infected the air above the earth and killed men in diverse parts of the world.

I can prove this conclusion by adducing some arguments in support that are taken from signs and circumstances that have occurred, of which the first is this:

It is well known that the mortality, as far as Germany is concerned, first began in Carinthia after an earthquake there, in which the vapor and air that was shut up in confined places in the mountains violently burst forth and hurled the highest mountains down into the subalpine valleys, destroyed the entire town of Villach, and buried very many of the mountain villages near the town of Arnoldstein. Then the same mortality advanced in succession into Austria, Hungary, Bavaria, Moravia, Bohemia, the Rhineland, Swabia and other German provinces, and now it invades Franconia. For it does not observe a regular order in its progress, but, as if blown by the wind, this unclean disease is conveyed now to one place, now to another, by a varying and irregular migration. So the cause that pertains to it does not seem to be easily assigned to anything else, except to the corrupt air, which has burst forth from the earth in an earthquake. . . .

For these and similar reasons, it seems to me that the cause of the said mortality was, and continues to be, the fact that the air was infected and poisoned by corrupt vapors and poisonous exhalations that were released and issued forth during earthquakes.[4] But against this position there are doubts, of which the first is:

That in some parts of the world, the said mortality began prior to there having been an earthquake. From this, it does not seem that an earthquake can be its cause.

The second doubt is that such a vapor, once it had been unleashed, would have soon dispersed and thinned out, so that henceforth it by no means would have harmed such a wide swath of people.

The third [doubt] is that the air in this way should be infected every time there is an earthquake, and thus a mortality of men would ensue after each earthquake. Yet this is not found in the chronicles or in scripture with regard to what they relate about what happened at the time.

---

[4]In his *Book of Nature*, Megenberg gives five reasons why he believes "the common death came from the poisoned air," including the observation that pears harvested at the time floated rather than sank in water, as they normally do, which Megenberg explained was because "the poisonous vapor ate them through and through as they drew a lot of air into themselves." See Megenberg, *Buch der Natur*, 134–35.

The fourth [doubt] is that when all the air is infected [by earthquakes], then everyone in their homes and villages should have died, which is not the case, since some have remained alive in these same homes and villages. . . .

I will answer these objections in plain language, [addressing] the principal reasoning behind each question.

To the first objection, which stated that in some parts of the world the mortality began prior to there having been an earthquake, I say that one must consider not only this very great earthquake that inflicted so much damage in Carinthia and in other parts of Germany, but also those [earthquakes] that occurred before and after in regions beyond the sea and in Italy and in Rome. And in this regard, I say that before that great earthquake happened, the spirits were held captive within the confines of the earth for so long that they pressed and forced themselves against the sides of the earth with the strongest pressure, because it was not easy for them to quickly topple so weighty a mass, and through this intensity of pressure not a little of the spirits or vapor steamed forth from the fissures in the earth and infected the air in some places.

To the second [doubt], it must be said that there was not a little of that earthly fume, which moved out over the length and breadth of the land, and not just one time or in one place only. For this reason, it could not have vanished and disappeared in so short a time, and concerning this [fume], even though we have experienced a diminishing of its impact over a long [distance], and it continues to disperse, nonetheless, no one can know exactly when it may disperse entirely, since a very great mortality still persists in some places in Germany, and in several other places it may begin for the first time.

To the third doubt, I say that it is not necessary that a mortality follow every earthquake and in every place where [an earthquake] has occurred, since, in accordance with the various dispositions of the earth, the spirits enclosed therein are affected and altered in various ways, so that one of [the earth's] contents changes another towards its own temperament, that is, towards its own disposition. And therefore, the spirits lurking in some of our mountains and in the recesses of some of our lands are more tainted with a foul corruption, and more afflicted with dispositions contrary to the fragile human condition, than in other lands. We see this in the case of water, where it yields up diverse tastes in accordance with how it resides in diverse lands, and some [waters] are potable, but others not so much.

To the fourth [doubt], I say that men have diverse complexions. For some are more compact and have a stronger resistance and are less susceptible [to disease], so that they do not easily succumb to anything foreign [to their bodies]. But others are the opposite: They have a delicate and soft constitution and easily succumb. And this is the reason why some die but others don't from the same causes. To this, one can add that [men follow] a variety of regimens during their lives. Hence we see that something that is food and nourishment for one man, is poison for another.

30

CITY AND COMMUNE OF PISTOIA

Ordinances

May 2, 1348, and May 23, 1348

Among the few civic ordinances to survive from the Middle Ages are those enacted by the city and commune of Pistoia in May 1348, about a month after the Black Death struck the city in March or April. Other Italian towns, such as Pistoia's neighbor, Florence, also enacted ordinances during the plague, but their full texts do not survive. Only those ordinances relating to the environment—specifically, the potential corruption of the air—are printed here, including revisions published on May 23, about three weeks after the original ordinances were proclaimed on May 2. The introduction to the ordinances notes that they were composed by "certain wise citizens of the city of Pistoia, chosen and deputed by the noblemen and by the gonfalonier of justice [that is, high magistrate] of the said city, with regard to preserving the health of the human body and correcting and resisting various and diverse pestilences that henceforth can be found in human bodies."

[May 2, 1348]

4. Item, they [i.e., the authors of these ordinances] provide and ordain that, in order to avoid the foul odor that is given off by the bodies of the dead, each grave in which any dead body is to be buried should be dug two and a half armlengths under ground, as this is reckoned in the city

A. Chiappelli, "Gli Ordinamenti Sanitari del Comune di Pistoia contro la Pestilenza del 1348," *Archivio Storico Italiano*, ser. 4, 20 (1887): 10, 12, 15, 17–18.

of Pistoia.[1] Penalty of 10 pence, to be paid by the gravedigger and also by whoever orders the grave to be dug, to be assessed on each offender and for each offense that infringes the statute.

5. Item, they provide and ordain that no one, of whatever condition, status, or standing, should dare or presume to bring and carry into the city of Pistoia any dead body, whether in a coffin or not, or in any other way. Penalty of 25 pence, to be paid by each offender carrying and bringing [such body], and by whoever arranges [for such body] to be carried and brought [into the city], to be paid for each offense. And the guards of the gates of the said city should not allow such a body to be brought into the said city, on penalty of the same to be paid by each man guarding the gate through which the said body was brought. . . .

13. Item, they provide and ordain that, in order that the bodies of the living not be sickened by putrid and spoiled food, no butcher or seller of meat, even in the smallest amounts, should dare or presume in any way to inflate meat [with a bellows], or to keep meat inflated,[2] or to sell, or arrange to have it kept and sold and inflated, in his shop or over the counter. Penalty of 10 pence, to be paid by each butcher and seller of meat and for each offense committed in the aforesaid manner. And the masters of the butchers' guild are bound for the time being to investigate and enquire concerning the aforesaid things on every day that meat is slaughtered, and they are to immediately denounce those found culpable to the lord *podestà* or *capitano* [i.e., high magistrates], or to one of their officials, under the aforesaid penalty, to be paid by the same masters, or by any one of them, if they or any one of the masters does not arrange for all of the aforesaid things to be carried out. And the *podestà* and *capitano* are each bound for the time being to send one of their officials to inspect and investigate and enquire concerning each and every one of the aforesaid things contained in this article [of the ordinance], and they are to fine and punish with the said penalty those found culpable and those masters, or any one of them, who does not at first denounce whoever committed the offense, as is stated above. And the word or report of any official who finds any transgression against the said statute is to stand and be believed, without any other proof being necessary. . . .

22. Item, in order that its stench and putridity cannot injure men, any tanning of skins cannot or ought not be done henceforth within the

---

[1]The grave must be between five and six feet deep; each *brachio* or armlength was equivalent to between two and two and a half feet.

[2]Medieval butchers would skin a carcass by inserting a bellows under the skin and inflating it with air, thus separating the skin from the flesh.

walls of the city of Pistoia.[3] Penalty of 25 pence to be paid by each man who performs the said tanning, and for each offense.

[Revisions of May 23, 1348]

Item, it is provided and ordained that, in a restating and correction of article 22 of these ordinances, which begins, "Item, in order that its stench and putridity, etc.," and that ends, "for each offense," should be added to, and the added words should be understood as thus, namely: That skinners and tanners of skins should be able, and it is allowed to them, to tan the skins that they have now in their tanneries in the usual manner, [which is to take effect] from the day of enactment of the present ordinance [i.e., May 23], until the 15th day of the month of June next to come. And moreover, that henceforth the tanning of skins may be done, and ought to and can be done, within the walls of the city of Pistoia, but only in the following places, namely: in the houses lining the street and *contrada* [district] from the courtyard or house of the canons of Pistoia situated in the chapel of Santa Maria del Nuova in the city of Pistoia, [then] down the street along which one goes towards the gate of San Pietro of the said city, up to and in the vicinity of the said gate, and including the land round about the said gate. And they may stretch out their skins and do other things necessary for the said tanning process, as it pleases them, in the aforesaid places. And [tanning] should be done, and ought to and can be done, in the place below the Castell Traiecti, up to and in the vicinity of the Carmelite friary of Santa Maria del Monte, and in the houses and courtyards and land situated in the said places. And anyone who goes against the aforesaid [stipulations], or against any one of them, is to be fined and punished for each offense, according to the penalty contained in this said article of the said ordinances.

Item, it is provided and ordained, in order that no putridity and stench can harm human bodies, that the rendering down of dripping or suet be done, or ought to be done, in a house or houses at least 25 armlengths [i.e., fifty to sixty feet] from other houses in the city of Pistoia, and not elsewhere. Penalty of 25 pence from each offender and for each offense.

Item, it is provided and ordained, that the tanning of gut, from which strings are made, is to be done, and ought to be done, outside the city of Pistoia, and not within the city itself. And the offender is to be fined and punished 25 pence for each offense.

---

[3]Medieval tanners removed the hair from the skins by soaking the skins in urine, and then softened them by soaking them in solutions of animal dung.

8

The Artistic Response

ST. SEBASTIAN AND ST. ROCH

Artistic images associated with the Black Death typically feature the *memento mori*, or macabre theme, in which a skeleton or decaying cadaver serves as a reminder of one's imminent death, a message that must have resonated all too well during a time of plague.[1] But more recently, scholars have been emphasizing the lighter side of death: that art with a thematic connection to plague can be optimistic, uplifting even, by incorporating themes of the afterlife or resurrection, when both the body and soul were meant to reunite and triumph over death, or even by raising the possibility that one could physically survive an attack of bubonic plague.[2]

Such is the case with the representation of the "plague saints," St. Sebastian and St. Roch. St. Sebastian, a Roman martyr who was executed by being shot by arrows and survived to be put to death a second time, is shown in fifteenth-century representations in a new guise, staring fixedly at the viewer just after his body has been pierced by multiple arrows from unseen executioners (Document 31). Even as the arrows symbolize the darts of pestilence, the clear message is that humankind can still triumph over the disease, just as Sebastian drew the arrows to his flesh in an act of Christ-like martyrdom, and yet survived.[3]

Likewise, St. Roch is depicted as a survivor, for him of plague itself. There is no mistaking this lesson, as Roch prominently displays the healed scar from a bubo on his groin or upper thigh, which, according to legend, he was able to cure through the aid of an "angelic doctor" and a faithful dog that carried bread to him during his illness (Documents 33 and 34). In some paintings, a twofold message is presented: that individuals can spare themselves the disease, even as others die all around them, by channeling the intercessory power of the saint through prayer; and that whole towns or communities can also be saved through the saint's ability "to wrest clemency from an angry God" and force Him to have "second thoughts" about exacting "punishment from a sinning humanity" (Documents 32 and 33).[4] In a time of disease and mass death, these messages must have held a powerful appeal, helping Europeans face, and ultimately overcome, the terror of the Black Death.

NOTES

[1] Paul Binski, *Medieval Death: Ritual and Representation* (Ithaca, N.Y.: Cornell University Press, 1996), 123–63.

[2] John Aberth, *From the Brink of the Apocalypse: Confronting Famine, War, Plague, and Death in the Later Middle Ages*, 2nd ed. (London: Routledge, 2010), 214–70.

[3] Louise Marshall, "Manipulating the Sacred: Image and Plague in Renaissance Italy," *Renaissance Quarterly* 47 (1994): 485–532.

[4] Ibid.

31

SANDRO BOTTICELLI

St. Sebastian

1474

Alessandro di Mariano di Vanni Filipepi, better known as Sandro Botticelli (ca. 1445–1510), was born in Florence and became one of the masters of the Early Renaissance. In 1474, he painted the tempera panel image of the martyrdom of St. Sebastian for the church of Santa Maria Maggiore in Florence. Note the way in which St. Sebastian gazes directly at the viewer, even as his body remains pierced with arrows.

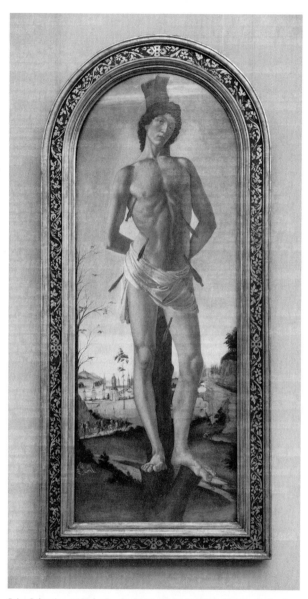

Saint Sebastian, 1474, by Sandro Botticelli (1445–1510) / Botticelli, Sandro
(Alessandro di Mariano di Vanni Filipepi) (1444/5–1510) / PRISMA
ARCHIVO FOTOGRAFICO (TARKER) / Gemaldegalerie, Staatliche
Museen zu Berlin, Germany / Bridgeman Images.

32

JOSSE LIEFERINXE

St. Sebastian Intercedes during the Plague in Pavia

ca. 1497–1499

Born in the diocese of Cambrai in Hainaut, which was ruled by the dukes of Burgundy (now the southern Netherlands), Josse Lieferinxe became active in the Provençal school of southern France. In 1497, he was commissioned by the Confraternity of St. Sebastian to paint an altarpiece dedicated to their patron saint in the church of Notre-Dame-des-Accoules in Marseilles, France. Lieferinxe chose as his subject the legend of St. Sebastian interceding with God to spare the city of Pavia during a plague outbreak there in the seventh century. Having never been to Italy, Lieferinxe based the appearance of Pavia on that of Avignon, whose architecture can be recognized in the background. Even as a victim collapses from a boil on his neck, the gravedigger, who wears a prayer slip to Sebastian just visible over the rim of his cap, remains unharmed.

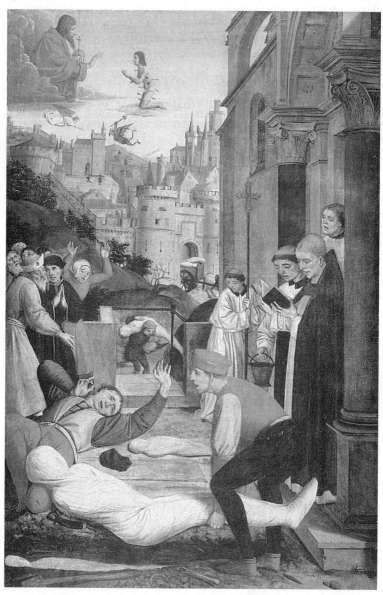

St. Sebastian Interceding for the Plague Stricken, 1497–99 (oil on panel) / Lieferinxe, Josse (Master of St. Sebastian) (fl. 1493–1508) / WALTERS ART MUSEUM / © Walters Art Museum, Baltimore, USA / Bridgeman Images.

33

BARTOLOMEO DELLA GATTA

St. Roch in front of the Fraternità dei Laici in Arezzo

ca. 1479

Born Pietro di Antonio Dei in Florence, Bartolomeo took his new name when he became a Camaldolese monk in 1468. Born in Florence in 1448, Bartolomeo della Gatta died in Arezzo, where he was abbot of San Clemente, in 1502. Around 1479, he painted a tempera panel image of St. Roch interceding with Christ before the lay fraternity of Arezzo, that Christ might spare the city from plague. On his right leg, Roch bears a scar from a plague bubo that has apparently healed.

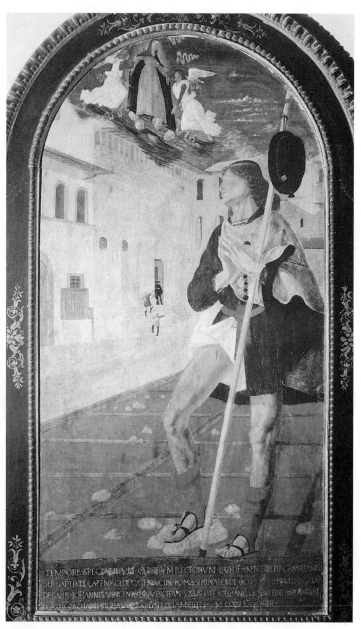

St. Roch in front of Lay Fraternity (Fraternità dei Laici) in Arezzo, by Bartolomeo
della Gatta (1448–1502), tempera on wood, 215 x 115 cm / DE AGOSTINI EDITORE /
Bridgeman Images.

34

German Woodcut of St. Roch

ca. 1480

This anonymous German woodcut of St. Roch depicts the typical features of his legend, including that an "angelic doctor" healed his bubo and that a dog fed him bread as he lay recovering in the woods.

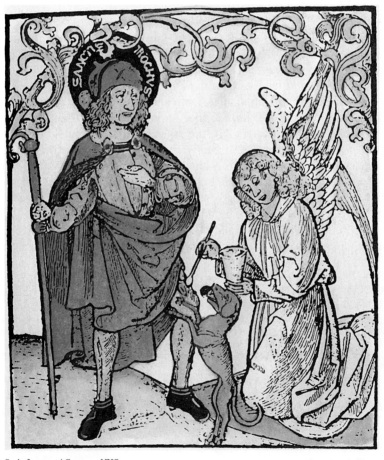

Sarin Images / Granger, NYC.

THE DANCE OF DEATH

The Dance of Death lends itself artistically to the experience of the Black Death for a number of reasons. As the great leveler, Death comes for all regardless of their position in the social hierarchy, just as plague made no distinctions in its onslaught on Europe's population.[5] In some versions of the dance, Death is a chess player, which seems to express the arbitrary and unpredictable nature of plague's geographical behavior. The chronicler Heinrich of Herford noticed this behavior, comparing plague's movements to "a game of chess."[6] In addition, a dancing Death, though frightening, is more approachable and familiar than the awesome figure of the Fourth Rider of the Apocalypse. Here, at least, a mortal can communicate with Death, before being taken away.

An elaboration on this theme is the late medieval English morality play *Everyman* (ca. 1485), in which Death appears at the beginning of the play to claim Everyman and lead him to his "reckoning." A long dialogue ensues, in which Death remains unmoved by Everyman's pleas for a delay of execution, until finally Death allows Everyman a brief respite to prepare his soul for the afterlife. As in John Lydgate's poem, *The Dance of Death* (Document 36), the afterlife in *Everyman* is described as a "pilgrimage," and Death comes regardless of rank or riches, setting naught "by pope, emperor, king, duke, nor princes."[7] But there is a revealing commentary at the end of the play in a monologue by Doctor, who points to the coming resurrection at the Last Judgment, when "we may live body and soul together."[8] The implied message that even a body rent by plague boils and other deformities will be fully restored at the end of time, finds a parallel in the Translator's introduction at the beginning of Lydgate's poem.

NOTES

[5]J. Brossollet, "L'Influence de la Peste du Moyen Âge sur le Theme de la Danse Macabre," *Pagine di storia della medicina* 13 (1969): 38–46; J. Batany, "Les 'Danses Macabres': Une Image en Negatif du Fonctionnalisme Social," in *Dies Illa: Death in the Middle Ages*, ed. J. H. M. Taylor (Liverpool: F. Cairns, 1984).

[6]Henricus de Hervordia, *Liber de Rebus Memorabilioribus sive Chronicon*, ed. Augustus Potthast (Göttingen: Dieterich, 1859), 280.

[7]*Everyman*, ll.126, 146.

[8]Ibid., 919.

The Great Chronicle of France

ca. 1348

The Great Chronicle *is a record of events of national importance kept by the monks of the abbey of Saint-Denis, where the kings of France were traditionally buried. According to the chronicle's editor, Jules Viard, this particular selection, which tells of people dancing to ward off plague in 1348, was probably written by an eyewitness who actually participated in the events described.*

In the year of grace 1348, the aforesaid mortality began in the kingdom of France and lasted for about a year and a half, more or less, and it was such that in Paris there died daily 800 persons. . . . And even though they died in such numbers, everyone received confession and their other sacraments. It happened that during the mortality, two monks from Saint-Denis rode into a town and were passing through it on a visitation at the command of their abbot. Thus they saw that the men and women of this town were dancing to the music of drums and bagpipes, and having a great celebration. So the monks asked them why they were making so merry, to which they replied: "We have seen our neighbors die and are seeing them die day after day, but since the mortality has in no way entered our town, we are not without hope that our festive mood will not allow it to come here, and this is the reason for why we are dancing." Then the monks left in order to go finish what had been entrusted to them. When they had accomplished their commission, they set out on the return journey and came back through the aforesaid town, but they found there very few people, and they had on very sad faces. The monks then asked them: "Where are the men and women who not long ago were holding such a great celebration in this town?" And they answered: "Alas! Good sirs, the wrath of God has descended upon us in the form of hail, for a great hailstorm fell upon us from the sky and came to this town and all around, and it came so unexpectedly that some were killed by it, and others died of fright, for they did not know where they should go or which way to turn."

Les grandes chroniques de France, ed. Jules Marie Édouard Viard, 10 vols. (Paris: Société de l'histoire de France, 1920–1953), 9:314–16.

JOHN LYDGATE

The Dance of Death

ca. 1430

A monk from Bury St. Edmunds in England, John Lydgate transcribed and translated the verses of the French poem of the Dance of Death at Les Innocents, apparently with the help of some native clerks, on a visit to Paris in the early 1430s, when the city was in English control. However, Lydgate introduced some variations that do not appear in the original French version, including references to the pestilence that appear in the stanzas printed in this selection. The first three stanzas are from the translator's introduction, a section that has no parallel in the French original. The last two are stanzas 53 and 54 from one widely accepted text of Lydgate's poem, in which Death dances with the Physician.

O yee folkes, harde herted as a stone
Which to the world have al your advertence [attention]
Like as hit sholde laste evere in oone [forever and anon]
Where ys youre witte, where ys youre providence
To see a-forne [in advance] the sodeyne vyolence
Of cruel dethe, that ben so wyse and sage
Whiche sleeth [slays] allas by stroke of pestilence
Bothe yonge and olde, of low and hie parage [station]. . . .

By exaumple that thei yn her ententis
Amende her life in everi maner age
The whiche daunce at seint Innocentis
Portreied is with al the surpluage [superfluities]
To schewe this world is but a pilgrimage
Geven unto us owre lyves to correcte
And to declare the fyne [end] of owre passage
Ryght anoon my stile [pen] I wille directe.

John Lydgate, *The Dance of Death*, ed. F. Warren and B. White (Early English Text Society, 181, 1931), 2–6, 52–54. By permission of Oxford University Press.

O creatures ye that ben resonable
The life desiringe whiche is eternal
Ye mai sene here doctryne ful notable
Yowre life to lede whiche that ys mortal
Ther be to lerne in [e]special
How ye schulle trace the daunce of machabre
To man and woman yliche [each is] natural
For dethe ne spareth hye ne lowe degre. . . .

Dethe to the Phisician:
Maister of phisik [medicine] whiche [o]n yowre uryne
So loke and gase and stare agenne the sunne[1]
For al yowre crafte and studie of medicyne
Al the practik and science that ye cunne [know]
Yowre lyves cours so ferforthe [far along] ys I-runne
Ageyne my myght yowre crafte mai not endure
For al the golde that ye therbi have wonne
Good leche [physician] is he that can hym self recure.

The Phecissian answereth:
Ful longe a-gon that I unto phesike
Sette my witte and my diligence
In speculatif [theory] and also in practike
To gete a name thurgh myn excellence
To fynde oute agens pestilence
Preservatifes to staunche hit and to fyne [cure it]
But I dar saie, shortli in sentence
Agens dethe is worth no medicyne.

---

[1]Examination of a patient's urine by color, smell, and even taste was a common diagnostic technique of medieval physicians.

TRANSI TOMBS

The transi tomb (from the Latin word *transire*, meaning to pass away) provided a variation on tomb monuments by substituting or contrasting a skeletal and rotting cadaver to the idealized, lifelike portrait of the patron. Nearly two hundred examples of transi tombs survive from northern Europe, particularly in France and England.[9] Transi tombs never seem to have been adopted in Mediterranean countries, perhaps because there custom decreed that the real corpse be on display during funerary ceremonies instead of being discreetly hidden away in a shroud or coffin.[10]

Interpretations of transi tombs typically have viewed them as the product of "a strong sense of anxiety about the fate of the soul [combined] with an intense preoccupation with death," to which the Black Death was undoubtedly a major contributing factor. In this view, the function of the transi tomb is to reconcile "the conflict between the growing worldly interests of the period and the traditional religious demand for humility."[11] It was not until the sixteenth century that the transi tomb supposedly came to symbolize a "new spirit" of the "triumph of worldly glory," despite the fact that the iconography remains essentially the same.[12]

A common feature of the transi tombs included here is a reference to worms. As a sign of corruption and decay, worms were closely associated with the Black Death. Yet here the worms may have an altogether different meaning, one that points toward the resurrection and restoration of the body, in line with the book of Job.[13] For example, it is possible to see the worms on the tomb of François de la Sarra as issuing *out* of the body, rather than crawling into it, symbolizing that the body is being restored to its original purity (Document 37). The presence of two scallop shells—ancient symbols of rebirth going back to the Greek myth of Aphrodite—that are depicted on François's pillow, one on either side of his head, strengthens such an interpretation. Similarly, one can "read" the double-decker transi tomb of Archbishop Henry Chichele, whose epitaph makes a couple of references to worms, in two ways: either downward, where the cadaver is the gruesome end product of decay of the resplendent effigy from above, or upward, where the upper effigy is now a resurrected body, accompanied by a host of heavenly angels, rising from the ashes of the corpse below (Document 38).

Perhaps the strongest affirmation of this theme comes from the mid-fifteenth-century English poem *A Disputacioun betwyx the Body and Wormes*. The *Disputacioun* is a dream vision by the poet, who in the opening lines establishes the setting for his poem: "In the ceson of huge mortalite / Of sondre disseses with the pestilence."[14] The debate envisioned in the poem between the female patron of the tomb and the worms that crawl through her dead body ends only with the body's realization that at the resurrection, it will finally triumph over death, corruption, and the worms. As the body says to the worms at the end of the poem:

> This that I hafe complened and sayd
> In no displesyng take it yow unto.
> Lat us be frendes at this sodayn brayde [outburst],
> Neghbours and luf as before we gan do.
> Let us kys and dwell to gedyr evermore,
> To that God wil that I sal again upryse
> At the day of dome [Last Judgment] before the Hye Justyse.[15]

NOTES

[9]A list of surviving transi tombs is included in Kathleen Cohen, *Metamorphosis of a Death Symbol: The Transi Tomb in the Late Middle Ages and the Renaissance* (Berkeley: University of California Press, 1973), 189–94. Note that Cohen does not include transi tombs in Ireland, which are discussed in H. M. Roe, "Cadaver Effigial Monuments in Ireland," *Journal of the Royal Society of Antiquaries of Ireland* 99 (1969): 1–19.

[10]Philippe Ariès, *The Hour of Our Death*, trans. Helen Weaver (New York: Oxford University Press, 1991), 114.

[11]Cohen, *Metamorphosis of a Death Symbol*, 48.

[12]Ibid., 120–81.

[13]Job 19:25–27 states: "For I know that my redeemer liveth, and that He shall stand at the latter day upon the earth; and though after my skin worms destroy this body, yet in my flesh shall I see God."

[14]For a more extensive discussion of the poem, see Aberth, *From the Brink of the Apocalypse*, 243–46; M. M. Malvern, "An Earnest 'Monyscyon' and '[Th]inge Delectabyll' Realized Verbally and Visually in 'A Disputacion betwyx [th]e Body and Wormes,' a Middle English Poem Inspired by Tomb Art and Northern Spirituality," *Viator* 13 (1982): 415–43.

[15]British Library, MS Add. 37049.

37

FRANÇOIS DE LA SARRA

Tomb at La Sarraz, Switzerland

ca. 1390

A leading nobleman from the Vaud region in present-day Switzerland, François de la Sarra served in various posts for his lord, Count Amedeo VI of Savoy, during the mid-fourteenth century. He died around 1363 and was buried in a chapel he founded with his wife, Marie, in his hometown of La Sarraz. On the basis of artistic influences, however, scholars favor dating the tomb to the 1390s, when it would have been erected by François's grandsons, rather than to the decade immediately after his death. The most prominent features of François's nude transi figure are the worms that crawl in or out of his arms and legs, and the frogs or toads that cover his eyes, lips, and genitalia. Two scallop shells were carved on the body's chest and two on the pillow on either side of his head, of which only one survives.

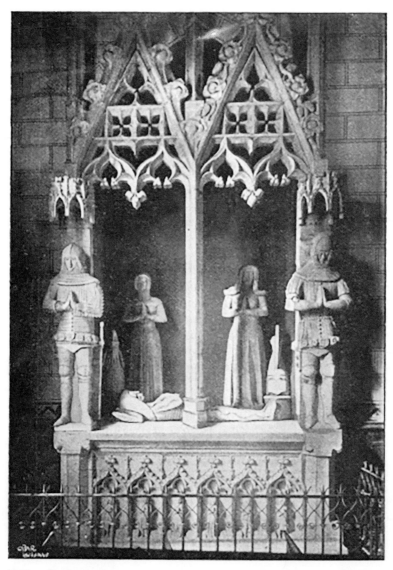

M. M. van Berchem.

38

ARCHBISHOP HENRY CHICHELE

Tomb at Canterbury Cathedral
ca. 1425

One of the most important churchmen and political figures in England during the first half of the fifteenth century, Henry Chichele was closely linked to his patron, King Henry V. In 1414, Chichele became archbishop of Canterbury, the most powerful churchman in the country. By 1425, less than three years after the untimely demise of Henry V in 1422 and nearly twenty years before his own death in 1443, Chichele had completed his transi tomb. The first such monument built in England, it started the trend of double-decker tombs. Chichele may have been inspired to make this kind of monument from the double image of effigy and coffin that was paraded at state funerals, including that of Henry V, or from witnessing the elaborate monument of Cardinal Jean de la Grange at Avignon (1402), a town Chichele no doubt visited in his capacity as an ambassador to France. Although no worms are depicted on Chichele's transi, worms feature prominently in the inscription of Latin rhyming couplets that runs around the lower border of the tomb surrounding the transi.

I was a pauper born, then to this primate [archbishopric] raised.
Now I am lain in the ground, ready to be food for worms.
Behold my tomb: 1442 [1443].
Whoever you be who will pass by, I ask you to remember,
You will be like me after you die,
For all [to see]: horrible, dust, worms, vile flesh.
May the assembly of saints unanimously intercede for him [Chichele],
So that God may be appeased by their merits on his behalf.

Kathleen Cohen, "The Changing Meaning of the Transi Tomb in Fifteenth- and Sixteenth-Century Europe" (Ph.D. diss., University of California, 1973), 652–53.

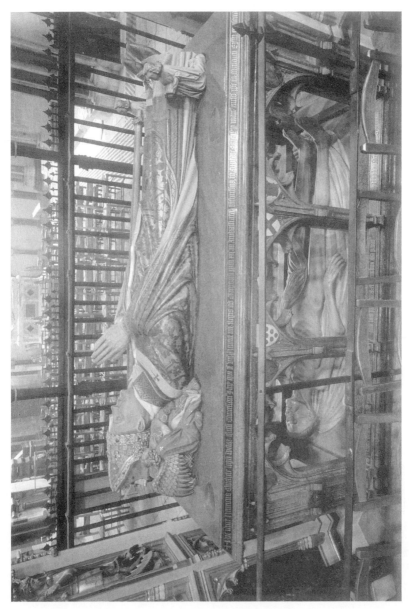

Angelo Hornak.

161

A Chronology of the Black Death
(1347–1363)

1347   Plague comes to the Black Sea region, Constantinople, Asia Minor, Sicily, Marseilles on the southeastern coast of France, and perhaps the Greek archipelago and Egypt.

1348   Plague comes to all of Italy, most of France, the eastern half of Spain, the coast of southern Spain, southern England, Switzerland, Austria, the Balkans and Greece, Egypt and North Africa, Palestine and Syria, and perhaps Denmark.

The flagellant movement begins in Austria or Hungary.

Jewish pogroms occur in Languedoc and Catalonia, and the first trials of Jews accused of well poisoning take place in Savoy.

1349   Plague comes to western Spain and Portugal, central and northern England, Wales, Ireland, southern Scotland, the Low Countries (Belgium and Holland), western and southern Germany, Hungary, Denmark, and Norway.

The flagellants progress through Germany and Flanders before they are suppressed by order of Pope Clement VI.

The burning of Jews on charges of well poisoning occurs in many German-speaking towns, including Strasbourg, Stuttgart, Constance, Basel, Zurich, Cologne, Mainz, and Speyer; in response, Pope Clement issues a bull to protect Jews.

Some city-states in Italy and the king's council in England pass labor legislation to control wages and ensure a supply of agricultural workers in the wake of plague mortality.

1350   Plague comes to eastern Germany and Prussia, northern Scotland, and all of Scandinavia (Denmark, Norway, Sweden).

King Philip VI of France orders the suppression of the flagellants in Flanders.

The córtes, or representative assembly, of Aragon passes labor legislation.

1351–
1352 Plague comes to Russia, Lithuania, and perhaps Poland.

The córtes of Castile, the parliament of England, and King John II of France pass labor legislation, but the córtes of Aragon revokes it.

1354 King John II of France passes labor legislation.

The Jews of Catalonia and Valencia draw up a *takkanoth*, or accord, with King Pedro IV of Aragon in order to obtain a bull of protection from Pope Innocent VI.

1358 Rise of the Jacquerie, a peasants' revolt, in France.

1361–
1363 Plague breaks out again in Europe.

Questions for Consideration

1. Where did the Black Death originate? How was it first communicated to Europeans?

2. How would you compare the description of Black Death symptoms by chroniclers like Louis Sanctus (Document 4) and John VI Kantakouzenos (Document 5), and by doctors like Abū Ja'far Ahmad Ibn Khātima (Document 6)?

3. What advice given by medieval physicians to ward off the Black Death seems to you to have been most beneficial? What was least effective, or even harmful?

4. How do you think the poison thesis developed by plague doctors like Alfonso de Córdoba (Document 8) and Gentile da Foligno (Document 9) contributed to the "poison conspiracy" against Jews and others?

5. What was the most important social response to the Black Death, according to the authors of Documents 11–13? Be sure to explain how each author addresses this question.

6. Who, precisely, enacted the economic legislation in Documents 14 and 15, and why? How else might these legislators have responded to the economic challenges posed by the plague? Based on the evidence in Document 16, how did laborers respond to this legislation, and how effective were the labor laws?

7. Did medieval Europeans lose their faith in God as a result of the Black Death? Defend your answer. Did their religious response have any practical effect? How well did the Church and its priesthood respond to this crisis (Documents 17–19)?

8. Compare the Christian and Muslim responses to the Black Death (Documents 17–21). How were they similar, and how were they different? What tensions did each community experience during the plague?

9. Compare the account of the flagellants according to the flagellant scroll (Document 22) with that according to the chronicle of Fritsche Closener (Document 23) and the sermon of Jean de Fayt (Document 24). How are they similar? How are they different? What are the advantages and disadvantages to each type of document?

10. What replies to the Strasbourg interrogatory about the poisoning conspiracy (Document 26) would seem to you to be most persuasive to contemporaries? Which would be least convincing?

11. How much of the medieval environmental explanation of the plague (Documents 28–29) may be attributable to human action and how much to nature? Do you think the environmental regulations enacted by cities like Pistoia (Document 30) had any effect in preventing spread of the disease?

12. Which artistic example (Documents 31–38) seems to you to best sum up the experience of the Black Death? Defend your answer.

Selected Bibliography

GENERAL WORKS

Aberth, John. *From the Brink of the Apocalypse: Confronting Famine, War, Plague, and Death in the Later Middle Ages*, 2nd ed. London: Routledge, 2010.

Biraben, Jean Noël. *Les hommes et la Peste en France et dans les pays européens et méditerranéens*. 2 vols. Paris: Mouton, 1975–1976.

Bowsky, William M., ed. *The Black Death: A Turning Point in History?* New York: Holt, Rinehart and Winston, 1971.

Byrne, Joseph Patrick. *The Black Death*. Westport, Conn.: Greenwood, 2004.

Cantor, Norman F. *In the Wake of the Plague: The Black Death and the World It Made*. New York: Free Press, 2001.

Cohn, Samuel K., Jr. "The Black Death: End of a Paradigm." *The American Historical Review* (2002): 703–38.

———. *The Black Death Transformed: Disease and Culture in Early Renaissance Europe*. London and New York: Arnold and Oxford University Press, 2002.

Dols, Michael W. *The Black Death in the Middle East*. Princeton, N.J.: Princeton University Press, 1977.

Gottfried, Robert S. *The Black Death: Natural and Human Disaster in Medieval Europe*. New York: Free Press, 1983.

Herlihy, David. *The Black Death and the Transformation of the West*. Edited by Samuel K. Cohn Jr. Cambridge, Mass.: Harvard University Press, 1997.

Kelley, John. *The Great Mortality: An Intimate History of the Black Death, the Most Devastating Plague of All Time*. New York: HarperCollins, 2005.

Martin, Sean. *The Black Death*. Edison, N.J.: Chartwell Books, 2007.

McNeill, William H. *Plagues and Peoples*. Garden City, N.Y.: Anchor Press/Doubleday, 1976.

Nutton, Vivian, ed. *Pestilential Complexities: Understanding Medieval Plague*. Medical History Supplement, 27, 2008.

Ormrod, W. Mark, and Phillip G. Lindley, eds. *The Black Death in England*. Stamford, Lincolnshire: Watkins, 1996.

Platt, Colin. *King Death: The Black Death and Its Aftermath in Late-Medieval England*. Toronto: University of Toronto Press, 1996.

Williman, Daniel, ed. *The Black Death: The Impact of the Fourteenth-Century Plague.* Binghamton, N.Y.: Center for Medieval and Early Renaissance Studies, 1982.

Zahler, Diane. *The Black Death.* Minneapolis, Minn.: Twenty-First Century Books, 2009.

Ziegler, Philip. *The Black Death,* 2nd ed. London: Penguin Books, 1998.

PLAGUE DEMOGRAPHY AND GEOGRAPHY

Aberth, John. "The Black Death in the Diocese of Ely: The Evidence of the Bishop's Register." *Journal of Medieval History* 21 (1995): 275–87.

Arthur, Paula. "The Black Death and Mortality: A Reassessment." In *Fourteenth Century England,* vol. 6. Edited by Chris Given-Wilson. Woodbridge, Suffolk: Boydell Press, 2010, 49–72.

Benedictow, Ole J. *The Black Death, 1346–1353: The Complete History.* Woodbridge, Suffolk: Boydell Press, 2004.

———. "*Yersinia pestis,* the Bacterium of Plague, Arose in East Asia: Did It Spread Westwards via the Silk Roads, the Chinese Maritime Expeditions of Zheng He or over the Vast Eurasian Populations of Sylvatic (Wild) Rodents?" *Journal of Asian History* 47 (2013): 1–31.

Carpentier, Élisabeth. "Autour de la Peste Noire: famines et épidémies dans l'histoire du XIVe siècle." *Annales: economies, sociétés, civilisation* 17 (1962): 1062–92.

Cui, Yujun, et al. "Historical Variations in Mutation Rate in an Epidemic Pathogen, *Yersinia pestis.*" *Proceedings of the National Academy of Sciences* 110 (2013): 578–82.

Davies, Richmond A. "The Effect of the Black Death on the Parish Priests of the Medieval Diocese of Coventry and Lichfield." *Bulletin of the Institute of Historical Research* 62 (1989): 85–90.

Derbes, Vincent. "De Mussis and the Great Plague of 1348: A Forgotten Episode of Bacteriological Warfare." *Journal of the American Medical Association* 196 (1966): 59–62.

Emery, R. W. "The Black Death of 1348 in Perpignan." *Speculum* 42 (1967): 611–23.

Gottfried, Robert S. *Epidemic Disease in Fifteenth-Century England: The Medical Response and the Demographic Consequences.* New Brunswick, N.J.: Rutgers University Press, 1978.

Gyug, Richard. "The Effects and Extent of the Black Death of 1348: New Evidence for Clerical Mortality in Barcelona." *Mediaeval Studies* 45 (1983): 385–98.

Hatcher, John. "Mortality in the Fifteenth Century: Some New Evidence." *Economic History Review,* 2nd ser., 39 (1986): 19–38.

Herlihy, David. "Population, Plague, and Social Change in Rural Pistoia, 1201–1430." *Economic History Review,* 2nd ser., 18 (1965): 225–44.

Morelli, Giovanna, et al. *"Yersinia pestis* Genome Sequencing Identifies Patterns of Global Phylogenetic Diversity." *Nature Genetics* 42 (2010): 1140–43.

Norris, John. "East or West? The Geographic Origin of the Black Death." *Bulletin of the History of Medicine* 51 (1977): 1–24. With replies by Michael Dols and John Norris in idem 52 (1978): 112–20.

BIOLOGICAL AND MEDICAL ASPECTS

Arrizabalaga, Jon. "Facing the Black Death: Perceptions and Reactions of University Medical Practitioners." In *Practical Medicine from Salerno to the Black Death.* Edited by L. García-Ballester, R. French, J. Arrizabalaga, and A. Cunningham. Cambridge: Cambridge University Press, 1994.

Benedictow, Ole J. *Plague in the Late Medieval Nordic Countries: Epidemiological Studies.* Oslo: Middelalderforlaget, 1992.

———. *What Disease Was Plague? On the Controversy over the Microbiological Identity of Plague Epidemics of the Past.* Leiden: Brill, 2010.

Bolton, J. L. "Looking for *Yersinia pestis*: Scientists, Historians and the Black Death." In *The Fifteenth Century, XII: Society in an Age of Plague.* Edited by Linda Clark and Carole Rawcliffe. Woodbridge, Suffolk: Boydell Press, 2013, 15–37.

Bos, Kirsten I., et al. "A Draft Genome of *Yersinia pestis* from Victims of the Black Death." *Nature* 478 (2011): 506–10.

Campbell, Anna Montgomery. *The Black Death and Men of Learning.* New York: Columbia University Press, 1931.

Carmichael, Ann G. *Plague and the Poor in Renaissance Florence.* Cambridge: Cambridge University Press, 1986.

———. "Bubonic Plague: The Black Death." In *Plague, Pox, and Pestilence.* Edited by Kenneth F. Kiple. London: Weidenfeld and Nicolson, 1997.

Cohn, Samuel K., Jr. "Epidemiology of the Black Death and Successive Waves of Plague." In *Pestilential Complexities: Understanding Medieval Plague.* Edited by Vivian Nutton. Medical History Supplement, 27, 2008, 74–100.

———. "The Historian and the Laboratory: The Black Death Disease." In *The Fifteenth Century, XII: Society in an Age of Plague.* Edited by Linda Clark and Carole Rawcliffe. Woodbridge, Suffolk: Boydell Press, 2013, 195–212.

Conrad, Lawrence I., Michael Neue, Vivian Nutton, Roy Porter, and Andrew Wear. *The Western Medical Tradition, 800 B.C. to A.D. 1800.* Cambridge: Cambridge University Press, 1995.

Crisciani, Chiara, and Michela Pereira. "Black Death and Golden Remedies: Some Remarks on Alchemy and the Plague." In *The Regulation of Evil: Social and Cultural Attitudes to Epidemics in the Late Middle Ages.* Edited by Agostino Paravicini Bagliani and Francesco Santi. Sismel: Edizioni del Galluzzo, 1998.

Drancourt, Michel, Gérard Aboudharam, Michel Signoli, Olivier Dutour, and Didier Raoult. "Detection of 400-Year-Old *Yersinia pestis* DNA in Human Dental Pulp: An Approach to the Diagnosis of Ancient Septicemia." *Proceedings of the National Academy of Science* 95 (1998): 12637–40.

———. "Molecular Identification of 'Suicide PCR' of *Yersinia pestis* as the Agent of the Medieval Black Death." *Proceedings of the National Academy of Science* 97 (2000): 12800–803.

Ell, Stephen R. "Interhuman Transmission of Medieval Plague." *Bulletin of the History of Medicine* 54 (1980): 497–510.

Grmek, Mirko D., ed. *Western Medical Thought from Antiquity to the Middle Ages.* Cambridge, Mass.: Harvard University Press, 1998.

Haensch, Stephanie, et al. "Distinct Clones of *Yersinia pestis* Caused the Black Death." *PLoS Pathogens* 6 (2010): online, e1001134.

Henderson, John. "The Black Death in Florence: Medical and Communal Responses." In *Death in Towns: Urban Responses to the Dying and the Dead, 100–1600.* Edited by Steven Bassett. London and New York: Leicester University Press, 1992.

Hirst, L. Fabian. *The Conquest of Plague: A Study of the Evolution of Epidemiology.* Oxford: Clarendon Press, 1953.

Lenski, Richard E. "Evolution of Plague Virulence." *Nature* 334 (1988): 473–74. See also the companion article by R. Rosqvist, M. Skurnik, and H. Wolf-Watz, "Increased Virulence of *Yersinia Pseudotuberculosis*," idem: 522–25.

Little, Lester K. "Plague Historians in Lab Coats." *Past and Present* 213 (2011): 267–90.

Schuenemann, Verena J., et al. "Targeted Enrichment of Ancient Pathogens Yielding the pPCP1 Plasmid of *Yersinia pestis* from Victims of the Black Death." *Proceedings of the National Academy of Sciences* 108 (2011): 746–52.

Scott, Susan, and Christopher J. Duncan. *Biology of Plagues: Evidence from Historical Populations.* Cambridge: Cambridge University Press, 2001.

Shrewsbury, J. F. D. *A History of Bubonic Plague in the British Isles.* Cambridge: Cambridge University Press, 1970.

Siraisi, Nancy G. *Medieval and Early Renaissance Medicine: An Introduction to Knowledge and Practice.* Chicago: University of Chicago Press, 1990.

Twigg, Graham. *The Black Death: A Biological Reappraisal.* New York: Schocken Books, 1984.

SOCIAL AND ECONOMIC ASPECTS

Bean, J. M. W. "The Black Death: The Crisis and Its Social and Economic Consequences." In *The Black Death: The Impact of the Fourteenth-Century Plague.* Edited by Daniel Williman. Binghamton, N.Y.: Center for Medieval and Early Renaissance Studies, 1982.

Blockmans, W. P. "The Social and Economic Effects of Plague in the Low Countries, 1349–1500." *Revue Belge de philologie et d'histoire* 58 (1980): 833–63.

Bolton, Jim. "'The World Upside Down': Plague as an Agent of Economic and Social Change." In *The Black Death in England*. Edited by W. M. Ormrod and Phillip G. Lindley. Stamford, Lincolnshire: Watkins, 1996.

Borsch, Stuart J. *The Black Death in Egypt and England: A Comparative Study*. Austin: University of Texas Press, 2005.

Bowsky, William. "The Impact of the Black Death upon Sienese Government and Society." *Speculum* 39 (1964): 1–34.

Campbell, Bruce M. S. *Before the Black Death: Studies in the "Crisis" of the Early Fourteenth Century*. Manchester: Manchester University Press, 1991.

Fryde, E. B. *Peasants and Landlords in Later Medieval England*. New York: St. Martin's Press, 1996.

Goldberg, P. J. P. *Women, Work, and Life Cycle in a Medieval Economy: Women in York and Yorkshire, c. 1300–1520*. Oxford: Oxford University Press, 1992.

Hatcher, John. *Plague, Population and the English Economy, 1348–1530*. London: Macmillan, 1977.

———. "England in the Aftermath of the Black Death." *Past and Present* 144 (1994): 3–35.

Herlihy, David. "Deaths, Marriages, Births, and the Tuscan Economy (ca. 1300–1550)." In *Population Patterns in the Past*. Edited by Ronald Demos Lee. New York: Academic Press, 1977.

Herlihy, David, and Christiane Klapisch-Zuber. *Tuscans and Their Families: A Study of the Florentine Catasto of 1427*. New Haven, Conn.: Yale University Press, 1985.

Kircher, Timothy. "Anxiety and Freedom in Boccaccio's History of the Plague of 1348." *Letteratura Italiana antica* 3 (2002): 319–57.

Klapisch-Zuber, Christiane. "Plague and Family Life." In *The New Cambridge Medieval History. Volume 6: c. 1300–c. 1415*. Edited by Michael Jones. Cambridge: Cambridge University Press, 2000.

Mate, Mavis E. *Daughters, Wives, and Widows after the Black Death: Women in Sussex, 1350–1535*. Woodbridge, Suffolk: Boydell and Brewer, 1998.

Penn, S. A. C., and Christopher Dyer. "Wages and Earnings in Late Medieval England: Evidence from the Enforcement of the Labour Laws." *Economic History Review*, 2nd ser., 43 (1990): 356–76.

Putnam, Bertha Haven. *The Enforcement of the Statutes of Labourers during the First Decade after the Black Death, 1349–1359*. New York: Columbia University Press, 1908.

Thompson, James Westfall. "The Aftermath of the Black Death and the Aftermath of the Great War." *American Journal of Sociology* 26 (1920–1921): 565–72.

RELIGIOUS MENTALITIES

Cohn, Samuel K., Jr. *The Cult of Remembrance and the Black Death: Six Renaissance Cities in Central Italy*. Baltimore: Johns Hopkins University Press, 1992.

————. "The Place of the Dead in Flanders and Tuscany: Towards a Comparative History of the Black Death." In *The Place of the Dead: Death and Remembrance in Late Medieval and Early Modern Europe*. Edited by Bruce Gordon and Peter Marshall. Cambridge: Cambridge University Press, 2000.

Delumeau, Jean. *Sin and Fear: The Emergence of a Western Guilt Culture, 13th–18th Centuries*. Translated by E. Nicholson. New York: St. Martin's Press, 1990.

Dohar, William J. *The Black Death and Pastoral Leadership: The Diocese of Hereford in the Fourteenth Century*. Philadelphia: University of Pennsylvania Press, 1995.

Dols, Michael W. "The Comparative Communal Responses to the Black Death in Muslim and Christian Societies." *Viator* 5 (1974): 269–87.

Harper-Bill, Christopher. "The English Church and English Religion after the Black Death." In *The Black Death in England*. Edited by W. Mark Ormrod and Phillip G. Lindley. Stamford, Lincolnshire: Watkins, 1996.

Lerner, Robert E. "The Black Death and Western European Eschatological Mentalities." In *The Black Death: The Impact of the Fourteenth-Century Plague*. Edited by Daniel Williman. Binghamton, N.Y.: Center for Medieval and Early Renaissance Studies, 1982.

Smoller, Laura A. "Plague and the Investigation of the Apocalypse." In *Last Things: Death and the Apocalypse in the Middle Ages*. Edited by Caroline Walker Bynum and Paul Freedman. Philadelphia: University of Pennsylvania Press, 2000.

Stearns, Justin K. *Infectious Ideas: Contagion in Premodern Islamic and Christian Thought in the Western Mediterranean*. Baltimore: Johns Hopkins University Press, 2011.

FLAGELLANTS

Colville, A. "Documents sur les Flagellants." *Histoire litteraire de la France* 37 (1938): 390–411.

Dickson, Gary. "The Flagellants of 1260 and the Crusades." *Journal of Medieval History* 15 (1989): 227–67.

Graus, Frantisek. *Pest, Geissler, Judenmorde: Das 14 Jahrhundert als Krisenzeit*. Göttingen: Vandenhoek and Ruprecht, 1987.

Henderson, John. "The Flagellant Movement and Flagellant Confraternities in Central Italy, 1260–1400." In *Religious Motivation: Biographical and Sociological Problems for the Church Historian*. Edited by Derek Baker. Oxford: Basil Blackwell, 1978.

Jansen-Sieben, Ria, and Hans van Dijk. "Un slaet u zeere doer Cristus eere! Het flagellantenritueel op een Middelnederlandse tekstrol." *Ons Geestelijk Erf* 77 (2003): 139–213.

Kieckhefer, Richard. "Radical Tendencies in the Flagellant Movement of the Mid-Fourteenth Century." *Journal of Medieval and Renaissance Studies* 4 (1974): 157–76.

JEWISH POGROMS

Breuer, M. "The 'Black Death' and Antisemitism." In *Antisemitism through the Ages*. Edited by S. Almog and translated by N. H. Reisner. Oxford and New York: Pergamon Press, 1988.

Chazan, Robert. *Medieval Stereotypes and Modern Antisemitism*. Berkeley and Los Angeles: University of California Press, 1997.

Cohen, J. *The Friars and the Jews: The Evolution of Medieval Anti-Judaism*. Ithaca, N.Y.: Cornell University Press, 1982.

Crémieux, A. "Les Juifs de Toulon au Moyen Age et le massacre du 13 Avril 1348." *Revue des études juives* 89–90 (1930–1931): 33–72, 43–64.

Foa, Anna. *The Jews of Europe after the Black Death*. Translated by Andrea Grover. Berkeley and Los Angeles: University of California Press, 2000.

Graus, Frantisek. *Pest, Geissler, Judenmorde: Das 14 Jahrhundert als Krisenzeit*. Göttingen: Vandenhoek and Ruprecht, 1987.

Guerchberg, Séraphine. "The Controversy over the Alleged Sowers of the Black Death in the Contemporary Treatises on Plague." In *Change in Medieval Society*. Edited by Sylvia L. Thrupp. New York: Meredith Publishing, 1964.

Katz, Stephen T. *The Holocaust in Historical Context. Volume 1: The Holocaust and Mass Death before the Modern Age*. New York: Oxford University Press, 1994.

Langmuir, Gavin I. *Toward a Definition of Antisemitism*. Berkeley and Los Angeles: University of California Press, 1990.

———. *History, Religion, and Antisemitism*. Berkeley and Los Angeles: University of California Press, 1990.

López de Meneses, Amada. "Una consecuencia de la Peste Negra en Cataluña: el pogrom de 1348." *Sefarad* 19 (1959): 92–131, 321–64.

Nirenberg, David. *Communities of Violence: Persecution of Minorities in the Middle Ages*. Princeton, N.J.: Princeton University Press, 1996.

Stow, Kenneth R. *Alienated Minority: The Jews of Medieval Latin Europe*. Cambridge, Mass.: Harvard University Press, 1992.

ARTISTIC ASPECTS

Ariès, Philippe. *The Hour of Our Death*. Translated by Helen Weaver. New York: Oxford University Press, 1991.

Batany, J. "Les 'Danses Macabres': une image en negatif du fonctionnalisme social." In *Dies Illa: Death in the Middle Ages*. Edited by J. H. M. Taylor. Liverpool: F. Cairns, 1984.

Binski, Paul. *Medieval Death: Ritual and Representation*. Ithaca, N.Y.: Cornell University Press, 1996.

Boeckl, Christine M. *Images of Plague and Pestilence: Iconography and Iconology*. Kirksville, Mo.: Truman State University Press, 2000.

Brossollet, J. "L'influence de la peste du Moyen-Age sur le theme de la Danse Macabre." *Pagine di storia della medicina* 13 (1969): 38–46.

Clark, James Midgley. *The Dance of Death in the Middle Ages and the Renaissance.* Glasgow: Jackson, 1950.

Cohen, Kathleen. *Metamorphosis of a Death Symbol: The Transi Tomb in the Later Middle Ages and the Renaissance.* Berkeley and Los Angeles: University of California Press, 1973.

Huizinga, Johan. *The Waning of the Middle Ages: A Study of the Forms of Life, Thought and Art in France and the Netherlands in the Dawn of the Renaissance.* Translated by Frederik Jan Hopman. London: E. Arnold and Co., 1924.

King, Pamela M. "The English Cadaver Tomb in the Late Fifteenth Century: Some Indications of a Lancastrian Connection." In *Dies Illa: Death in the Middle Ages.* Edited by J. H. M. Taylor. Liverpool: F. Cairns, 1984.

—————. "The Cadaver Tomb in England: Novel Manifestations of an Old Idea." *Church Monuments: Journal of the Church Monuments Society* 5 (1990): 26–38.

Kurtz, Leonard Paul. *The Dance of Death and the Macabre Spirit in European Literature.* New York: Columbia University Press, 1934.

Marshall, Louise. "Manipulating the Sacred: Image and Plague in Renaissance Italy." *Renaissance Quarterly* 3 (1994): 485–532.

Meiss, Millard. *Painting in Florence and Siena after the Black Death: The Arts, Religion, and Society in the Mid-Fourteenth Century.* Princeton, N.J.: Princeton University Press, 1951.

Panofsky, Erwin. *Tomb Sculpture: Four Lectures on Its Changing Aspects from Ancient Egypt to Bernini.* New York: Harry N. Abrams, 1956.

Polzer, Joseph. "Aspects of the Fourteenth-Century Iconography of Death and the Plague." In *The Black Death: The Impact of the Fourteenth-Century Plague.* Edited by Daniel Williman. Binghamton, N.Y.: Center for Medieval and Early Renaissance Studies, 1982.

Rosenfeld, Helmut. *Der Mittelalterliche Totentanz: Entstehung, Entwicklung, Bedeutung.* Münster: Böhlau, 1954.

Saugnieux, J. *Les Danses Macabres de France et d'Espagne et leurs prolongements littérraires.* Paris: Belles Lettres, 1972.

Tristram, Philippa. *Figures of Life and Death in Medieval English Literature.* New York: New York University Press, 1976.

Van Os, H. W. "The Black Death and Sienese Painting: A Problem of Interpretation." *Art History* 4 (1981): 237–49.

POISON CONSPIRACY

Colet, Anna, et al. "The Black Death and Its Consequences for the Jewish Community in Tàrrega: Lessons from History and Archaeology." In *Pandemic Disease in the Medieval World: Rethinking the Black Death.* Edited by Monica Green. *The Medieval Globe* 1 (2014): 63–96.

Ritzmann, Iris. "Judenmord als Folge des 'Schwarzen Todes': Ein medizinhistorischer Mythos?" *Medizin, Gesellschaft und Geschichte* 17 (1998): 101–30.

Index

abandonment
  of family, 57, 58n1, 64–65
  of property, 64, 68, 69
abscesses, 32
Agramont, Jacme d', 47n1
  "Regimen of Protection against Epidemics,"
    52–56
agricultural workers, 57–58, 70, 72–78, 163, 164
air
  disease and, 27, 34, 42–45, 47, 49, 52–53
  earthquakes' effect on, 138–40
  pollution, ordinances on, 141–43
  stagnant air in wells, 138, 138n2
Airs, Waters, and Places (Hippocrates), 138n1
animals
  abandonment of, 68
  dying of plague, 22–23
  foretelling plague, 133
  spread of disease and, 2, 5, 7–8, 15n33, 15n37,
    15n39–40, 19, 27, 27n2
Annalium Hiberniae Chronicon (*Yearly Chronicle
  of Ireland*), 10
apocalypse, 5, 11, 19, 93
apostemes (tumors), 30
Aragon, kingdom of, 74
archaeology
  paleomicrobiology, 5–6, 9–10, 14n25, 28, 134
  rat bones and, 8, 15n37, 134n8
archbishops of Canterbury, 84–86, 160, 161f
Aristotle, *Concerning the Causes of the Properties
  of the Elements*, 42, 42n2
Armleder massacres, 124n6
artificial cause of disease, 46–47. *See also* poison
  conspiracy
artistic response to plague, 144–45
  paintings, 145–50f
  poetry, 24–25, 94–100, 154–57, 160
  tombs, 156–60, 159f, 161f
  woodcuts, 151, 151f
'Asqalānī, Ibn Hajar al-, 80
assize court roll, 76–78
astrology
  bloodletting and, 54–55
  cause of disease and, 41–46, 48, 53, 114, 136–37
  predictions from, 111
autopsy of bodies, 29, 30, 48, 56
Avicenna. *See* Ibn Sīnā

bacteria, 41. *See also Yersinia pestis* bacterium
bathing, 45, 55
bedding, 34–35
beggars, 75, 111–12, 130
"Beginning and End: On History, The" (Kathīr),
  88–90
behavior changes, 63–68

Benedict, André, "Letter to the Jurors of Gerona,"
  113–14
Berthold of Bucheck (bishop), 105
Bible
  apocalypse and, 11, 19
  flagellants and, 110
  Job, on death, 156, 157n13
  poison conspiracy and, 129, 129n1, 131n4
biological warfare, 135
Black Death. *See also* bubonic plague; pneumonic
  plague; septicemic plague
  arrival in Europe, 1, 19, 20f, 163
  denial controversy, 5–10, 13n15, 14n28–30, 134
  DNA testing for, 6, 13–14n21, 134n7
  economic impacts of, 57–59, 72–73
  geographical origins of, 19–27, 20f, 21n4
  historical significance of, vii–viii, 3–5
  history of, 1–3
  immunity to disease and, 32, 35, 140–41
  medical care, 40–41, 46–47, 49–50, 50n5, 51n6,
    54, 64
  medieval sources of information on, 10–11 (*see
    also specific sources*)
  positive effects of, 4
  prevention of, 46–47, 49–51, 50n5, 51n6, 52–56,
    64
  religious views of, 79–80
  social impacts of, 57–59
  survivors of, 5, 9, 32, 35, 140–41
  symptoms of, 28–39
  transmission of, 28–30
  types of plague, 9, 15n33, 29–30, 37–39
Black Death: A Turning Point in History?, The
  (Bowsky), 3
Blasius of Barcelona, 9
bleeding as remedy, 49, 49n4, 54–55
blood samples, 6
Boccaccio, Giovanni, 10, 57, 58n1
  Decameron, The, 57
bole, Armenian (clay), 51, 51n6
Bolton, J. L., 14n25, 14n30
Book of Nature (Megenberg), 136, 138n3, 139n4
Botticelli, Sandro, "St. Sebastian," 145, 146f
Bowsky, William, *Black Death: A Turning Point in
  History?, The*, 3
Bradwardine, Thomas (archbishop of Canterbury),
  84
buboes (lymph node swellings), 9, 34, 36, 37, 38,
  134n8
bubonic plague, 9, 29–30, 37–38. *See also* Black
  Death
Bukhārī, *Traditions*, 88, 88n1
burials. *See also* transi tombs
  death rate and, 3
  funerals, 57, 65–69